Your *Best* Birth

Your *Best* Birth

Know All Your Options,
Discover the Natural Choices,
and Take Back the Birth Experience

Ricki Lake
and
Abby Epstein

Foreword by Jacques Moritz, OB-GYN

**WELLNESS
CENTRAL**

NEW YORK   BOSTON

Some material has been adapted or reprinted from the following sources and is used with permission:
The Labor Progress Handbook, by Penny Simpkin and Ruth Ancheta, © 2005
Gayle Peterson, PhD, *An Easier Childbirth*, Shadow and Light Publications, © 1993
Victoria Macioce-Stumpf, www.choicesinchildbirth.com
Marsden Wagner, *Creating Your Birth Plan*, © 2006

Wellness Central
Hachette Book Group
237 Park Avenue
New York, NY 10017

Visit our Web site at www.HachetteBookGroup.com.

Wellness Central is an imprint of Grand Central Publishing.
The Wellness Central name and logo are trademarks of Hachette Book Group, Inc.

Printed in the United States of America

First Edition: May 2009
10 9 8 7 6 5 4 3 2 1

Library of Congress Cataloging-in-Publication Data
Lake, Ricki.
    Your best birth : know all your options, discover the natural choices, and take back the birth experience / Ricki Lake and Abby Epstein.—1st ed.
        p. cm.
    ISBN 978-0-446-53813-8
    1. Childbirth—Popular works. 2. Natural childbirth—Popular works. 3. Obstetricians—Popular works. 4. Midwives—Popular works. I. Epstein, Abby. II. Title.

RG525.L25 2009
618.2—dc22
                                                            2008046751

For our sons, Milo, Owen, and Matteo

Contents

Section Three

INTERVENTIONS: THE SLIPPERY SLOPE   115

Section Four

TAKE BACK YOUR BIRTH   167

Foreword

Jacques Moritz, OB-GYN

*Director of Gynecology at St. Luke's–Roosevelt Hospital and
Assistant Clinical Professor of Obstetrics and Gynecology,
Columbia University College of Physicians and Surgeons*

On a recent, beautiful fall day in New York City, my family and I went
for a walk around Gramercy Park. It was a walk we had taken a hundred times before, but this time, as we passed by a brownstone, we all
noticed a National Parks Foundation sign that read "The Birth Place
of Theodore Roosevelt." My fourteen-year-old son asked if Theodore
Roosevelt was actually born in this house or if it was just the place where
he grew up. I thought it was a great question. Of course the year, 1858,
meant that he was actually born in this house. My daughter's response
was "cool!" At that time, Mrs. Roosevelt didn't have a choice. Giving
birth at home was her only option.

A lot has changed in the 150 years since Mrs. Roosevelt delivered.
If you were to walk into the coincidentally named Roosevelt Hospital's
labor and delivery floor, where I'm the director of the gynecology division, the first thing you would see is two sixty-inch plasma monitors
displaying an array of data such as fetal heart rate, intrauterine pressure
readings, blood pressure, pulse oximetry readings, and the list goes on.
In front of these monitors would be a group of well-minded physicians
and nurses that are all "managing" the laboring women. It reminds me
of air traffic controllers at JFK trying to get a 747 on the ground in one

piece. And patients love it. They say, "The care must be good—look at all that high-tech equipment they are using." But is all this high tech a good thing? Have we now entered the day of "high-tech, low-touch" deliveries? And if we have, what are the risks and benefits? These are all questions that expecting mothers should ask themselves. These questions and more are answered in *Your Best Birth*.

In 2006, I was approached by Abby Epstein and Ricki Lake to be involved in a documentary for television that was initially titled, "Manhattan Midwives." I'm not a midwife but I am supportive of the midwifery model of care and have been the midwifery backup at Roosevelt Hospital for the past fifteen years. In fact, my own children were delivered by midwives. As Ricki and Abby began doing research for the film, they realized that they might have stumbled on a bigger question, How are babies born in the United States? What started as a film on midwives turned into *The Business of Being Born*, a film that became the childbirth equivalent of Al Gore's environmental exposé, *An Inconvenient Truth*. Birth, something that happens every day in America, was examined and questioned like never before.

Women and, especially, men have applauded at every screening, always saying the film opened their eyes to the many different ways you can have a baby. At the same time, after screenings at my hospital (where the film was actually shot) the film was being booed, with Abby and Ricki being called Nazi propaganda filmmakers. I remember going to Labor and Delivery just after the film was shown and a young OB running up to me in her full "space suit" (gown, booties up to knee, and a mask covering her entire face) looking like she had just come out of some biohazard, screaming, "You're not the only one that can deliver a baby naturally!" I had to chuckle. The most recent form of criticism came from the American Medical Association, which came out with an article announcing their stance that all home births were unsafe. I had never been aware that a film could be so powerful.

The state of obstetrics in America is in a crisis mode. The word "crisis" is a strong one that is overused in this country, but the obstetrical crisis is real. Women must understand this crisis and how it will affect their birth options. Physicians and midwives are being squeezed between the dual constraints of rising malpractice premiums and increasing law-suits. The record numbers of OB-GYNs who are voluntarily stopping obstetric practice and of midwives who are unable to find backup physicians or get malpractice insurance are signs of a major crisis. Even more importantly, there are increasing limitations imposed by insurance companies that introduce restrictions on how OBs can practice. In Oklahoma, for example, OBs are not covered by their malpractice provider for VBAC. Even if the doctor wants to provide a patient with the VBAC option, the hospital won't allow it because the hospital doesn't have the insurance coverage. Of course, in the classic "Catch 22" the insurance providers tell doctors that they can still do VBACs (vaginal birth after cesarean)—they just won't be covered. Obstetrics training itself is questionable, in my opinion. In my four years of residency at Columbia University, the only natural childbirth I ever saw was done by midwives.

The days of pregnant women interviewing their doctor (as seen in the film Knocked Up) may be a thing of the past. I know doctors who now interview patients to see if they will accept them in their practice, or "fire" patients if they have too many questions. The days of your health care provider's being the person who attends your birth are also over. Most OBs and midwives now practice in groups. Not a bad idea in theory, since the last thing a woman wants is someone who hasn't slept in the past forty-eight hours delivering her child. However, when it comes to today's common "mega" groups of OBs where you have eight OBs covering each other in a group, it means you have a one in eight chance of getting your doctor for delivery. And this new trend goes one step further with the "laborist," a physician who is now commonly hired by a hospital or large obstetrical group exclusively to deliver babies. Laborists often have twelve-hour shifts. You will never meet the laborist before you start labor and you won't see the laborist again after delivery, and if your labor is a long one, you may have more than one laborist taking care of you. Welcome to the new world of obstetrics.

When women find out they are pregnant, they're often so excited that the only thing on their mind is maintaining a healthy pregnancy. I understand, but the next priority should be deciding what kind of birth they desire. The first step in the process is finding the right health care provider, but there is information you need to know up front as you make this decision, and there are many more decisions that will follow. Do you want an OB or a midwife? What services are available in your local community? Is there a birthing center in your local hospital? Are you a good candidate for a birthing center birth? These are all questions that should be answered early on.

Most pregnant women run to the bookstore and leave with a stack of pregnancy books that briefly cover delivery in a short chapter at the end of the book, when it should actually be talked about in great detail early on. It's unrealistic to decide what kind of delivery you want in the last three weeks of pregnancy. The classic example is when a woman comes to her OB with a birth plan and finds out that her OB has different plans for her birth. I can't tell you how many times I get phone calls from women thirty-five to thirty-six weeks into pregnancy who are in disagreement with their OBs over their birth plans and want to transfer to a new doctor. Of course, I can't accept a patient at thirty-five weeks. I feel for these women because they are now in an antagonistic position with their health care provider. The outcome is sure to be a disappointment for all parties involved.

Thanks to Ricki and Abby, with *Your Best Birth*, women will have the opportunity to know more about the birthing landscape and how best to maneuver in it with the aim of having the kind of birth that's right for them. Although our health care system does not place the top priority on expectant mothers, you can still make the choices that will allow you to plan and prepare for your best birth. Maybe you are sure from the beginning that you want an epidural, or even an elective C-section. Those choices are yours. This book presents the risks and benefits of each. Abby and Ricki are internationally known advocates of informed choice, educating and empowering women at a moment when health care providers can't or won't present women with all of their viable options. It is up to you to discover your own options so that you can be your own advocate.

Above all, the goal is a healthy mother and healthy baby. As you'll come to find out in this book, how you arrive at that outcome is up to you. My hope and expectation is that *Your Best Birth* will lead you there.

Preface
Ricki and Abby: Our Best Births

Ricki

My pregnancies were miraculous times in my life. I felt special and very beautiful. I was also completely open to other people's suggestions. There isn't any other way to explain how a pharmacist's daughter was attracted to natural childbirth. Honestly, I'm a wimp. I like pain medication. I like my Tylenol with codeine for a headache. I like a sleeping pill once in a while too. Yet when I was pregnant with my first child, I talked to a friend of mine, a woman who never had so much as an aspirin during labor, and what she said sounded good to me. Being pregnant isn't being sick. So it made sense that, as a healthy twenty-seven-year-old woman, I wouldn't need to be medicated to bring my baby into the world. The point was, as she described it, to feel everything. Feel *everything*? Most of us expend a lot of energy trying not to feel. No, she said, in this the goal was complete surrender.

I'm a Virgo, and we grip on to things pretty tight. In labor, supposedly, the best part comes when you give yourself over completely to these uncontrollable sensations. My friend Ana Paula Markel, who is a doula (personal labor assistant), describes labor as a struggle to find a balance between control and surrender. That's not just labor, that's most women's lives. Surrendering to this with my child would bond us forever, no matter what troubles we faced up the road.

My friend referred me to a midwifery practice that worked in part-nership with a hospital birth center. I loved all the attention they lavished on me. When I went for my prenatal visits, we talked about everything: nutrition, fears, exercise, my feelings about my body, my relationships with my mom and with my husband. Part prenatal care, part therapy. Midwives say that with an obstetrician you spend an hour in the wait-ing room and five minutes with the doctor. With a midwife you spend five minutes waiting and an hour with her. After nine months of this, I really trusted my midwife.

The birth center took up part of a floor of St. Luke's–Roosevelt Hos-pital in New York City. When Abby saw it later, she thought the big birthing tub and the blocky, impersonal furniture made it feel like a cheesy hot tub suite in a slightly run-down Las Vegas hotel. The sheets on my bed at home had a much higher thread count.

At the time, I thought it was beautiful. Right then, though, I thought everything was beautiful. Even my 210-pound ass was beautiful to me. Besides, it didn't appear that having the baby there would in any way be a gamble. The labor and delivery department was on the next floor if anything went wrong. Since this was my first baby, I wasn't sure how much pain this wimp could handle. They assured my husband and me that at the birth center all the choices would be ours.

As my due date approached, I was probably the happiest and most serene I'd ever been, joyful about welcoming our little boy into the world, confident that my husband and I had made all the right choices. I also wanted this baby when I wanted it. I had three weeks off from work and I anticipated his arrival that first weekend. Fortunately he agreed. My water broke early on the morning of my due date. My contractions were far apart, not very powerful, and not escalating. I thought the baby was just taking his time, coming when he needed to come. When we got to twenty-four hours without much happening, Sandy, my midwife, said it was time for us to come to the birth center.

When we got there, Sandy told us we had only four hours to get my labor going or they would have to start me on drugs. Twenty-four hours after a woman's membranes rupture, the hospital requires the staff to speed up labor because they fear she will get an infection. The hospital has a timetable (called protocols) that the doctors and midwives follow strictly. If they don't, there may be legal consequences. My husband, Rob, and I walked the halls, but not much changed. After a few hours of that, we decided we needed to take more drastic action. He held my hand as we climbed up and down the stairs, feeling the pressure of time mounting as the minutes ticked by. I was getting more and more upset. I could see a C-section looming on the horizon. That was the last thing I wanted.

By the twenty-eight-hour mark my midwife said that we needed to get this labor going. I wanted to resist, but I didn't want to be selfish. The most important thing was to have a healthy baby. The rules had to be written with that in mind. Still I was sobbing as Rob held my hand and we took the stairs from the birth center to the labor and delivery floor.

They started me on Pitocin, a drug that stimulates contractions. Once the Pitocin was in, I couldn't move about as freely because I was dragging the IV pole. They also put an internal fetal monitor in my baby's scalp so they could see how he reacted to the contractions. Powered by Pitocin, the contractions were really slamming me. They call these contractions "camelback" because they are two-humped, one right after the other. They gave me Stadol, a drug that was supposed to take the edge off my feelings of despair, but it affected me horribly. I panicked. I kept saying to Rob, "Is something wrong? I feel like something is going wrong." The pain was unbearable.

I needed an epidural, a steady drip of painkillers that block the transmission of pain up the spine, so I could get some rest between contractions. The pharmacist's daughter welcomed that. The anesthesiologist got the dosage just right, thank God. He blocked the pain, but I could still feel my feet, which allowed me to squat when I pushed. Still I couldn't escape my panic no matter how much reassurance I got. I didn't want anyone from the hospital staff to touch me then. I didn't trust anyone but Rob. Every decision made to get me on the hospital's schedule took away a bit of what we wanted for this birth.

In the end, though, I pushed for two and a half hours and out came Milo, beautiful and healthy. Most women don't really want to dwell on their birth experiences. You get this amazing gift of the baby. You're on a high and whatever happened in the hospital just seems to fade away. Even if it didn't go as planned, it was a pretty amazing experience. I feel blessed that, considering it all, I had a vaginal birth for my first child. And although Rob and I are now divorced, the memory of how he was on that day is one of the things I can draw on when I need a little encouragement to get over one of our postmarital spats.

When the mommy-bonding hormones stopped coursing through my veins, I started to think about the birth, not just the baby. How quickly everything had changed direction. At the hospital, I felt like a problem. I wasn't progressing fast enough, they said, even though my baby was never in distress. I remembered how when my mom came to see us at the hospital, I introduced her to my midwife saying, "Mom, here's the woman who delivered my baby!" Sandy corrected me, "Ricki, you're the one who delivered that baby." Why couldn't I shake this feeling that my body had betrayed me?

Hadn't this crazy system betrayed me? Keeping my prenatal appointments, eating my green, leafy vegetables, the vitamins, the yoga, the visualizations—all of it built a sense that this would be a birth of my own creation. After so many months of preparation, in the end I never had a chance to surrender except to the hospital's schedule. I was never in control. I had wanted to feel everything, but all I remembered of labor was fear and panic. I had blocked out the glory of pushing my baby into the world so much that I gave Sandy credit for delivering Milo. Why the big disconnect? Suddenly I was very interested in birth.

I became a birth junkie. Two months after Milo was born, I started going to birth conferences. I wasn't planning to have another child right away, but I wanted to educate myself. I read everything. I never studied like this in school. Back then I never cared enough about what I was learning. For a little while I got it in my head that I wanted to be a midwife. It's my calling, you know? When I told my family and friends, they thought I was insane. They pointed out this wasn't realistic for a talk show host who hadn't managed to get an undergraduate degree.

Nutty, I know, but it shows how much birthing Milo opened up my world. This country makes mothers feel so bad, so inadequate, even at the moment of the births of their babies. Yet everybody at the birth conferences was so pro-mother and pro-baby, and the conferences were so much about honoring them and fighting this uphill battle against what has been happening in for-profit childbirth. I began to believe (and I've had a lot of arguments with people about this) that how they are born affects who babies are. I realized the process was so important to me. If I were to have another child, I wanted to do it my way. I wanted to have the people around me that I felt comfortable with. I wanted to be in an environment where I felt completely safe and at home. And I didn't want my baby taken away from me. I didn't want any intervention that wasn't necessary. I felt that I could only have it my way by doing it at home.

Five years later, when I was pregnant again, I met Miriam Schwartzchild, a midwife with a really great reputation in the home birth world. We connected. I was comfortable with her protocols. I told her my goal was to have a positive experience and to remember everything—every contraction, every position, every feeling. Miriam completely understood my desire to have a water birth at home. She was so relaxed, as if this was not a big deal. I loved that she came to my home for my prenatal care. We'd drink tea and talk while Milo came in and out and asked his own questions. A friendship grew. By the time I went into labor, I was so comfortable with her. There was no question that this was what I should be doing.

I was eight days from my due date when my water broke early in the morning as I sat on the toilet. It happened to be the first day of Milo's very first summer day camp. It was so amazing to think that he was going off to camp and chances were pretty good that he would be coming back to meet his new brother. My doulas came to our apartment first and Miriam came around eleven o'clock. In the early stages of labor we played Scrabble. We sat on the floor and I would take breaks between contractions. We were about to choose letters to begin another round when I had to stop because my labor started to move pretty quickly. Just at the moment when I had picked a blank, the ultimate letter, I had to quit!

I got to know every corner of my apartment that day. I positioned myself in every room of my house: on the floor, in the bathroom, throughout the hallway. There were moments, many moments toward the end, when I thought I couldn't do it. The phase they call "transition," when I was going from seven to ten centimeters, was the most challenging time. That's when you're not fucking around anymore. You're dead serious and you're in pain. I remember specifically being at the sink in my kitchen, my chin resting on the waterspout, and thinking, "I cannot do this anymore." I heard an ambulance go by and I said, "There's my ride. Get me out of here."

Miriam looked me in the eye and reminded me of the reasons I chose to be at home in the first place. I needed someone to tell me I was right and this was right and exactly what Rob and I wanted. After that, I surrendered to it. When I did that 100 percent, things moved very quickly. Shortly after that, the head started coming out. Miriam said if I wanted to have my baby in the water like we had discussed, I had to get in the tub right away. In the tub, I pushed for thirteen minutes, three contractions. Then Miriam told me to reach down and touch my baby. I placed him on my chest and he stared right at me with his eyes wide open.

We got out of the tub and into the bed. They talk about the high you have with a natural childbirth. It's so true. I had all this energy. I mean, I was flying. I was so psyched. I wasn't tired at all. My whole labor was nine hours start to finish. Right after, I was on the phone calling everyone and having food delivered, having friends over. I did all of this as Owen nestled in my arms nursing. After nine months of sharing my smell, voice, and heartbeat with him, I didn't want him even two inches away from me. Only after two hours did Miriam ask if she could check him over and weigh him.

It was so huge. I still can't believe I did it. And it's not just what my body did in giving birth; it's that I went against so many people around me. I chose to go against much of the advice given to me, went the opposite way and did what I wanted, and it turned out even better than I expected. No one can take that away from me. I also think I gave Owen a gift. I did something for him that will affect him no matter who he is. I'm grateful and hope he'll grow up to be grateful for that too.

I admit that so far neither one of my boys has taken me aside to thank me for his birth. At least neither of them has ever said that he is sorry he was born. Not yet anyway. I love both of my boys so powerfully that the words I can summon up to describe that love sound puny by comparison. How Owen was born is part of the many things I love about him, but I don't love Milo any less. I love them and their births that brought them to me, but I also love how giving birth to them allowed me to grow as a woman.

With Milo, I planned as carefully as I could, but the experience was wrenched out of my hands. I organized Owen's birth much differently, with a different kind of support that allowed us more intimacy and more control. Even when you don't have much control, as the birth of Abby's son, Matteo, shows, you can still make it a beautiful and fully supported experience. When Abby became a mother, she started from a different place and went through a much different experience than I did with either of my sons' births.

Abby

A lot of women approach birth with a certain vision and a passion. I had no vision at all. Or excitement for that matter. I always knew I wanted to have children, but the actual birth process seemed pretty unappealing to me, pregnancy included. Before Ricki and I started working on *The Business of Being Born*, our film about childbirth, I really only knew about traditional hospital birth. No one in my family ever went to a midwife. I thought midwives were hippies with no medical training whose ignorance might endanger you or your baby.

Although I generally do not like hospitals, I instinctively felt that having an epidural was the way to go because it would give me more control over the situation and would allow me to be calm and present, instead of a screaming, raving lunatic. I really wasn't interested in birthing, which always looked so scary and disgusting on television. Thirty hours in labor? There's nothing about me that would ever want to embrace pain. Why would you put yourself through that? I would have been like, "Hello, I'll take an epidural now." I didn't have anything to prove to anyone, including myself. Like most mothers-to-be, my goal was just to have a healthy baby.

After nearly two years of filming the documentary together, my partner, Paulo, and I decided that we were going to try getting pregnant. I didn't think my birth would become part of the film because I suspected it would take forever to conceive. It seemed like all the women I knew in their mid-thirties were having fertility issues. I thought it would take a year, at least. But we got pregnant on the first try. I was in shock. Suddenly I had to think about what kind of birth we wanted.

When I was only a few weeks pregnant, we filmed our first home birth. It was the first live birth that I had ever witnessed and it was magical. We drove up to Harlem with the midwife in the middle of the night and baby Naima was born in a birthing pool in the middle of the living room as the sun came up. We ordered in breakfast from a local diner and celebrated with the new family. From that time on, everything shifted. We continued to follow this home birth midwife, Cara Muhl- hahn, who became a character in our film, and we were so impressed with the way she straddled the spiritual and medical aspects of birth, as well as being an excellent clinician.

I didn't know if I would be more comfortable in a hospital birth center or at home. Initially, there were some issues with my HMO because none of the hospital-based midwifery practices accepted my insurance plan. So I started out seeing an obstetrician, Dr. Jacques Moritz, who supported all my options and I decided to stay with him until we were through all the "testing" phases and then seek out new insurance that would be accepted by a midwife. Dr. Moritz is also known around New York as the "hairy midwife," so I knew we would be in good hands. When I was thirty weeks pregnant, we decided to go for the home birth with Cara and Dr. Moritz offered to act as our "backup" doctor. I felt comfortable with Cara and trusted that she was competent. I truly didn't see the advantage of being in the birth center over being at home. As far as the safety profile went, being in Manhattan, there were so many hospitals nearby, including one a few minutes from where we lived.

I had a really easy pregnancy except that every exam confirmed the baby was breech, meaning butt down instead of head down. A breech baby would prevent us from having a home birth and would mean a scheduled cesarean section. At about thirty-five weeks, I was waiting for my third appointment with Cara to discuss trying some of the options to reposition the baby: acupuncture; chiropractic; and moxibustion, where burning herbs are rubbed on your pinkie toe. Sounds a little out there, but I researched it. Apparently some acupuncturists who are skilled at moxibustion have a 50 percent success rate. Also the baby wasn't that big. I knew he still had some room, so I hadn't given up hope. We didn't even get to that point, though.

That weekend, I woke up with some weird cramping in my groin and I didn't feel the baby moving as much. Cara told me to be sure that the baby moved every time I ate. She suggested that if I was concerned about decreased fetal movement, I could go to the hospital and have a nonstress test to check out the baby. I did feel some movement after I ate and I believed he was okay. I didn't go to the hospital.

The next day, we were shooting all day at a medical panel called "Seeking the Perfect Baby through C-Section." Ricki was in town and we were going to meet that evening for a margarita. (She would be the only one indulging, of course.) But by nine o'clock, I felt wiped out and told Ricki I couldn't make it. Paulo and I were lying on the couch when I started having light contractions every five minutes. I didn't think anything of it until I went to the bathroom and saw a spot of blood. I called Cara. As soon as Cara heard that there was "show," she said she was coming over to check on me. She told me to get in the tub and have a glass of wine or beer because alcohol can slow down contractions. I got into the tub but couldn't drink; the alcohol made me nauseous.

I had no idea that I could seriously be in labor. All the first-time labors we'd filmed were epic in length, and most of the women were at least a week late delivering. I was due July 12 but imagined that I'd give birth closer to July 22. It was only June 14. My family was leaving the next morning for a weeklong bike trip in Europe they had planned specifically so that they would be back in time for the birth. I kept thinking maybe I should call them to make sure they didn't go to the airport. Cara said I shouldn't call them until we knew what was going on.

When Cara arrived, she gave me that Cara look. Midwives are always trying to smell if you're in labor. She started assembling all the information. She checked the heartbeat and found that the baby was doing great. She checked his position and determined that he was still breech. She said we should look at my sonogram.

There was a chance that if the baby was near enough to term, we could turn him and have a vaginal birth. Cara has had success doing that, but it can't be done if the baby's too early. We looked at the date and other signs and confirmed that I was at thirty-five and a half weeks. We all knew that we were not going to attempt a breech delivery at home, and the baby's early arrival added a second complication.

Cara checked me while I was lying in bed—I was dilated to four centimeters. I was in total shock. None of us could believe it was happening. I was just so, so, so unprepared. No diapers, no baby stuff. I had no crib. Ricki rushed over to be my doula. Cara said we needed to go to the hospital right away because she didn't want to take a chance that my water might break at home. While Paulo threw a bunch of things into our big red duffle bag, Cara called Dr. Moritz to tell him that we were heading to the hospital. I felt so bad she had to wake him up in the middle of the night.

Usually Cara drives her car to every birth so that she has it handy in case of a transfer to the hospital. Since she lives only a few blocks from us, she had just walked over with her birth kit. The car service she called was taking forever, so she grabbed a taxi.

I was not too happy in the cab. The labor really started to pick up as we sped toward the hospital, which was on the opposite side of the city. Cara asked if I preferred to go to a closer hospital, but I really wanted Dr. Moritz to be there. I trusted that if there were any possible way to turn this baby, he would try it, even though I knew the chances were slim to none at this point. Ricki held me through all the contractions in the taxi and Cara monitored the baby's heartbeat with a Doppler. Paulo sat in the front seat filming (yes, we were still making our documentary!) and trying to keep the cab driver calm as I screamed at him to go through the red lights. I could feel this baby was dropping down and coming fast. My water broke just as we were stepping out of the taxi.

When we got up to labor and delivery, it was like the SWAT team descended. The staff was shouting, "Get a monitor on her! Get an IV!"

Cara handed the staff my file and medical history. I was on the exam table on my hands and knees having a contraction when they put papers in front of me to sign. I said, "Can you just wait until this contraction is over?" Paulo tried to pull the papers away to take some control. One nurse stuck an IV in my hand and another nurse wrapped a belt on me while somebody else came in and said, "Hi, I'm a resident and I'm going to check you," followed by "Okay, she's six." All of a sudden, I started hearing myself talked about in the third person. I realized the whole situation was now out of our hands.

Soon I was in the operating room on my hands and knees on top of the table. A resident gave me a shot in my leg to slow down the labor while we waited for Dr. Moritz to arrive. I didn't feel any more contractions after that. A kind woman who introduced herself as the midwife on call checked me again. She said that I was fully dilated and the baby was "right there" so she would do a vaginal breech delivery since this was my third child. As much as I loved the idea of delivering this baby, I informed her that this was actually my *first* child. The anesthesiologist asked the midwife to leave so she could begin my spinal.

By the time Dr. Moritz arrived, I was completely calm and joked with him that we really had left for the hospital promptly and did not intend to have such a dramatic arrival.

Cara held my hand and described what Dr. Moritz was doing throughout the surgery. For me, the C-section birth was completely surreal. Some people who have a vaginal birth say that it's also surreal. I feel that there's something about pushing a child out of your body, whether you feel it or not, and touching your baby immediately that makes it real.

All I could feel was this strange nausea from the anesthesia and then Dr. Moritz saying, "Easy...easy...cord around the neck...Okay, we got him." I heard the nurse say, "He's a little peanut." I didn't understand that meant he was very small. There was a long silence before he started crying, and, since I couldn't see anything, I began to panic. After they cleaned him up, the nurse brought him around the table to give me a quick peek. He looked catatonic. I remember thinking, "Oh, my God—is he autistic? What's the matter with him? He looks weird. He looks stunned." The nurse whisked him off to the neonatal intensive care unit (NICU) and I didn't see him again for more than twenty-four hours.

Luckily Paulo got to go into the NICU right after Matteo was born and put him on his chest for some skin-to-skin contact. I didn't have that maternal desire to be with my baby like I thought I would. I was on too many drugs, too groggy. I was dying of thirst, but the nurses wouldn't let me drink. During the four hours I spent in the recovery room, I couldn't even imagine holding a baby. I was shivering uncontrollably as the anesthesia wore off. My mom was freaking out. Then I was moved from recovery into a temporary hospital room until there was a room available for me. Next to my bed, I had a Polaroid snapshot one of the nurses had taken of my baby. He was so tiny with a full head of hair. All I could do was stare at that little picture. I was so out of it. Looking back, I see that I was, in fact, post-traumatic.

The next day, the nurses removed my catheter and told me that Paulo could wheel me down to the intensive care unit to see my baby. I still felt that I didn't want him to meet his mother when I felt so miserable, drugged up, and in so much pain. I remember Paulo pushing me down the hall in my wheelchair and seeing all these other new moms doing the "C-section shuffle." They waddled down to the nursery all hunched over their incisions, taking little baby steps and dragging their IV poles. When I saw Matteo for the first time, it was a very emotional moment. He was so tiny and had many wires attached to his little body. They said he probably couldn't breast-feed, but he did. I was lucky and thankful that my breasts filled with milk right away.

We found out that Matteo had experienced something called intrauterine growth restriction in the womb (IUGR). Probably somewhere between thirty-two and thirty-five weeks, either there was too much compression on the cord and his nutrients were cut off or there might have been some sort of a breakdown in the placenta. The doctor said that his head was slightly bigger than his body, a sign that more of the nutrients were shunted to the brain. I am sure that's also part of the reason why he went into early labor. He was developed enough to survive outside on his own. He was small, but his lungs were fine. I believe that there is an inherent wisdom in nature's design. In the end, I thought, "My God, I'm so lucky." Although it wasn't what we'd planned, everything worked out okay. Matteo started the labor and came out at the right time for him.

For months after Matteo was born, I felt disconnected from his birth. I felt as if I were the victim of a car crash instead of a glowing new mother. Cara helped me process all of this. She made me the hero of my story in a way. She made me see myself as an active protagonist. For any woman who has had an emergency C-section, it's a good way to look at it. You're not helpless. Even though you may not feel like you had a normal childbirth experience, it is a birth that should not be discredited. I had to credit myself for assembling a great birth team and putting myself in a situation where we did get to the hospital on time.

Although the dash to the hospital and the emergency C-section were traumatic, I never felt Matteo and I were in any real danger or that my little birth team of Cara, Ricki, and Paulo couldn't handle the situation. In truth, I really did feel empowered. I had information and wasn't going to do anything unknowingly or be railroaded into a certain kind of birth. I surrendered to the birth Matteo needed, and I don't feel disappointed. I think it's almost impossible, in that moment when you have a new baby, to feel disappointed about anything. In some ways, it was a perfect entry into parenthood—these little people arrive and make their own path beyond your control. They start teaching you lessons before they are even born.

Ricki and Abby

Pregnant women reading our very different birth stories have probably had some pretty strong reactions to the circumstances we created and the decisions we made. Some decisions you might disagree with. There are things we dismissed, times we hesitated, and aspects we downplayed that you would have done differently. "Oh my God, I'd never have a home birth," some might think. "That's just too risky." Others might think that Abby was right in the beginning: Sign me up for the epidural and the hospital, no looking back. Abby's cab ride alone is enough to make many women gasp. We sure were gasping.

That's why we told our stories in such detail. Not only did we want to show you that we've been through it, all of it in its various twists and turns, but we also wanted to get you thinking about what would be the best birth for you and your baby.

Some say that even when women are old and senile, even when they have trouble recognizing old friends, they can still remember the days their children were born in vivid detail. How you are treated and how you cope are things that stick with you for the rest of your life. What happens on that day can connect you more strongly to the world and to those you love, or it can reinforce everything you loathe and fear about yourself and the world around you. In this way, it's too important to take passively or unconsciously, or to leave in the hands of strangers. Birth, like life, is full of surprises. When Abby says it is a perfect introduction to motherhood, what she means is that you plan and dream, compromise and compensate, and, in the end, your child will probably have a slightly different idea about all of it.

So even though you can't predict, you can prepare. You can get to know your body, understand your fears, strengths, and values, and get familiar with how the medical world might react to all of that and all of you. This book is an attempt to put in your hands all of what we didn't know when we started to consider the births of our children so that you can give your life with your baby a good start by arranging the best birth possible.

Introduction

Your Birth Is Your Business

Let's say right up front that we are not writing a book that tells you that you should birth your baby in a particular way. Honestly, it's none of our business what you do. We're not experts, except in the way that any woman who has given birth is an expert. Women have a lot of choices when they consider the births of their children and each of those choices has passionate advocates.

There are people who say you are an idiot if you birth any place but a hospital, and there is a zealous minority who warn that, given our country's alarming C-section rate, you're taking a huge risk unless you birth at home. It seems simple and obvious to say that a woman should have the kind of birth that suits her body, her baby, and her level of anxiety. This could mean having your baby at the hospital with a midwife and a doula at your side, at a birth center, or at home—maybe even a water birth. It could even mean a scheduled C-section. It's your baby, after all.

What we're going to show you in this book is how, because this is your baby, it's up to you to decide what kind of birth is best for you—even if it's different from the type your sister, cousin, or best friend had. It could even be a type of birth that your own OB-GYN hasn't initially suggested to you. Your best birth is one where you feel empowered because you know all your options and are confident in the decisions you have made about the birth.

These days it is simply not enough to "trust your doctor." The birthing world is filled with distrust and litigation so you need to listen to your own instincts. We believe that women intuitively know what is best for themselves and their unborn babies and that listening to this inner voice during your pregnancy is preparation for motherhood.

In addition to taking responsibility for your labor and birth, at the end of the day you also need to surrender control. Babies come on their own time and in their own way—they dictate how and when they need to be born. The most important outcome is a healthy mom and a healthy baby. That's a given. It's not about whether you had the most tranquil, painless water birth in your rooftop Jacuzzi (yes, we've heard that story!) or had to be completely knocked out for an emergency C-section.

Neither experience will affect how much you love your child. But we believe that you can place the health and well-being of your newborn as your highest priority and still have an optimal, empowering experience that is right for you both—whether that is in your bed, in your bathtub, in a hospital room, or on an operating table. All the choices are yours and we want to give you some information and encouragement to resist and question the current trend toward more medicalized births that are not appropriate for everybody.

We know that figuring those things out is a lot to consider at a time when you're tired, grouchy, and dealing with a body that is behaving in unfamiliar ways, so we're going to guide you through this. The purpose of this book is to help you explore the full spectrum of choices you have in giving birth. And most importantly, to make you feel confident that you not only have considered all of your options but also understand the many circumstances beyond those decisions that affect the process. Considering what women are up against, every birth is heroic.

So what are you up against?

You're up against a whole lot of knowledge and a whole lot of ignorance. There are huge obstetrical textbooks, most more than a thousand pages thick, that describe everything science knows about birth. Equally large books could be written about what the medical community doesn't know. If doctors had a better understanding of how labor starts, they'd do a much better job at induction and at delaying premature birth. Yet we tend to cede a lot of our power to the doctors. Most Americans believe that, with doctors in charge, decisions will be impartial and made with the mother's and the baby's best interest in mind. But that's far from certain in many decisions made on the labor and delivery floor.

For example, when you're in labor and they lay you on the hospital bed with your feet in the stirrups, the way 67 percent of American women give birth, they're actually slowing your labor down. Lying on your back closes the pelvis by 25 to 30 percent, and in that position gravity no longer works in your favor. These counterintuitive practices might be acceptable if they were improving our outcomes, but the United States has some of the highest infant and maternal mortality rates in the developed world, scraping the bottom of the list alongside Cuba. Our C-section rate is closing in on a third of all deliveries, twice what the World Health Organization says is safest for mothers and babies. Many of these C-sections are not medically necessary, and are done simply out of convenience or fear of malpractice suits.

You'd think with all the scientific innovations and specialized equipment available to mothers in this country that American women would have the world's safest, most trouble-free births. Instead, fear increasingly dominates birth. Women have been taught that being in labor might be too hard and too painful and to be focused on its dangers. Despite the wisdom of the natural processes of our bodies, we're taught that we are powerless to some extent. The technology developed to help the doctors understand what is going on inside the womb during the birth—such as the fetal monitor—in many ways has removed maternal confidence and dulled the instincts women have relied upon for centuries when giving birth.

When our documentary on this subject, *The Business of Being Born*, premiered in January 2008, we were overwhelmed by the response we received at screenings. Some doctors like to dismiss women who advocate natural childbirth as elitists and crackpots; yet, in city after city, the screenings were packed with women from all walks of life, all segments of the economy, many of whom were holding their babies on their hips or chasing them down the theater aisles when they stood up at the question and answer period after the film to tell their birth stories. In the telling of these passionate, heroic stories (some of which you'll read in these pages), some women shook with rage and several broke down in tears. Many had gone to extraordinary lengths to achieve the kind of birth they wanted: traveling great distances, driving full speed in the dead of the night. One woman who had previously had a C-section labored in the parking lot of a hospital so that she'd be admitted too far dilated for anyone to refuse her a vaginal delivery.

When we heard these stories, we thought about how brave these mothers were and how incredibly determined they had to be to get what they wanted in a system that is so far out of whack. These were women who, just like any good mother, were trying to act in the best interest of their children but were faced with lawyers and hospital conglomerates that narrowed their birthing choices simply to shield practitioners from lawsuits and to fatten the corporate bottom lines. Many of these women told us that afterwards they wished they had been aware of the choices they had in giving birth.

There is a lot of information about giving birth on the Web and many books written by respected academics and experienced caregivers who have unearthed and examined America's strange and sometimes horrifying birth practices in exhaustive detail. So exhaustive, in fact, that those books are sometimes a little hard to read. Which is why—politics aside—this information isn't as widely known as it should be. What the women we met at our screenings wanted was a book that would demystify the natural options that their doctors didn't present as viable—and that would offer these options in a straightforward and comprehensive format that could educate and *empower* women. This is that book.

In this book we will be looking to a wide array of experts to educate you about the possibilities that generally don't come up in discussions with doctors and in hospitals. That amazing day when your baby is born will be one that lives in your memory for the rest of your life and the lives of everyone who shares it with you. It is also a day when you are under an extraordinary amount of pressure. Some of the situations women find themselves in, and some of the decisions they are pressured to make, might be very different if they understood how politics and economics combine with physiology to influence their choices.

As you may already know, there is a certain stigma attached to natural childbirth. Many people think it's something that only hippies and hardcore feminists would consider—not to mention masochists who thrive on pain. What doesn't generally get discussed is that childbirth isn't always as painful as it looks on television, and that you can actually overcome the pain during contractions using your own inherent strength. What really doesn't get discussed is the adrenaline rush that can power you through labor, and the high that often follows natural childbirth. Some women even say that this high makes it all worth it.

A funny thing happens when women start talking about natural childbirth. At first it can sound totally unappealing. But when a woman starts to learn all the ins and outs, and begins to understand why so many women are choosing this path, she may find herself creating a new birth plan that she previously never would have imagined. Take one of the women we photographed for the cover of this book. After hearing about our birth experiences, she changed her doctor and birth plan immediately—just one week before her due date!

We will tell the stories of many births in this book, what women planned for, which of those plans worked out, and how they themselves were transformed as a result. As we said, if you end up needing a C-section, we want you to feel confident and informed about the decision. If you've educated yourself and understand why your doctor says this is what needs to happen, you won't be second-guessing him or her or feel you've consented under pressure. The goal is to feel that you are part of the decision-making process—not that your doctor is dictating and you're just along for the ride. We encourage you to consider the advice in this book and to discuss it with your medical professional.

Intermixed with the tales of everyday moms, we're going to sprinkle in the stories of well-known women like Cindy Crawford, Kellie Martin, Melissa Joan Hart, and Laila Ali, who had their babies naturally. Recently celebrities who scheduled elective cesareans have gotten a lot of attention in the media. We think that those who took a different path and chose a natural childbirth should be noted too, to show you that a more natural birth is not as "out there" as some have been led to believe.

This book is not intended to lecture you about the way you should have your baby, but is about helping you overcome your fears, the pressures, and the fads and ultimately allowing you to have an empowering and beautiful experience to share with your family. This book will serve as a reminder that giving birth is something that women instinctually know how to do, and that you can tap into your own innate sense of power to take back the birth experience.

Your *Best* Birth

KNOW YOUR OPTIONS

What kind of birth do you want?

Dare to think, just for a moment, that you could actually get the kind of birth that exactly suits your needs, the needs of your baby, and your desires. What would it look like? Where would you be? Who would you have around to support you when things got tough? Would you want something for the pain right away? Or would you like to give birth without drugs? And in those precious moments after your baby takes his or her first breath, is that child resting on your chest? Or being examined by a doctor to make sure that everything is okay? If you close your eyes and piece together all the different elements, what sequence of events would make you happiest and most secure?

Considering how unquestioning most of us are about the inevitability of giving birth the American way, it's hard to know where to start in creating a birth of your own design. Where do you start to ask questions? Who do you ask them of? The place to start is with you.

For generations back everybody in your family has had their babies in the hospital, most likely. When your friends and your relatives go to the hospital to give birth, you don't see what happens there. (For many decades, even fathers weren't allowed in maternity wards.) You only see the result: your loved one propped up in bed holding that scrunchy-faced little newborn. The baby is the focus of most of the anxiety and most of the attention after the birth, so your experience of the hospital recedes quickly into the background. We're going to tell you what the typical hospital birth is like for the mom because we expect no one has ever described it to you.

We need to say up front that we're talking in a general way and trying to go right down the middle in terms of what most hospitals offer. You might live in a place where the hospital is extremely accommodating and caters to even the most fussy demands of pregnant moms. Or you might have as your advocate a very powerful doctor or midwife who, by force of personality and reputation, gets great treatment for all of her patients. It's even more likely that your hospital offers a lot of good things, some flexible policies and practices, and some routine procedures that are not very friendly to the way you want to deliver your child.

Any description we offer here will miss some of the specifics of the hospitals in your area because every one, every state, every staff is different. So why bother describing? There are some things that are generally true and knowing them now, before we get to the finer points of the decisions you will be making for yourself and your baby, will give you a working knowledge of the way birth is managed in America. So we'll start with you, the general you, as you enter the hospital in labor.

In this hypothetical scenario, you've been in labor since early in the morning but the contractions are weak and disorganized. You call your doctor's office when it opens and the nurse tells you to call back when the contractions are consistently five minutes apart and much stronger. Some time after dinner, the pace starts to pick up and they get stronger. When you page your doctor around eight in the evening, the doctor on call, a doctor unfamiliar to you, tells you to go to the hospital.

The hospital's main entrance is closed, so you enter through the emergency room. The staff directs you to the elevators that will take you to the maternity ward. When you enter the maternity ward, they put you in the triage room, a big room with four beds, two of which have other women in different stages of labor. All of you are being evaluated to see if you should be admitted, and your partner is told to wait in the hallway. Suddenly alone, you are separated by curtains and can hear the other women clearly as the nurses look you over. The nurses hand you a big pile of documents to fill out.

Before you get on the bed to be examined, you see the fetal heart rate monitor, with its stretchy wide belt made of fabric that is much like a girdle but shaped like a tube top. Monitoring in triage is a hospital requirement to get an initial reading on the baby's heart rate. The nurse points you to the bathroom and tells you to give them a urine sample, after which you have to put on the fetal heart rate girdle.

The nurse places a glove on her hand and inserts her fingers in your vagina to determine how soft and wide your cervix is and how far your baby has progressed. Her assessment of these two things determines that you are three centimeters dilated, far enough along to stay. For a first-time mom, few hospitals will admit you unless you are at least that dilated. As the heart rate monitor gives out its readings, the lab is testing your urine to see if you have any kidney problems. The nurse also checks your vital signs: temperature, blood pressure, pulse, and breathing.

It is a busy night in the maternity ward and you have to stay in the triage room for a while waiting for a room to open up and be cleaned. While you wait, you address all the forms that need your signature. There are a lot of things to specify including allergies and drug sensitivities as well as consent forms for different procedures including anesthesiology. This is a very hurried and stressful time as you absorb this new atmosphere, the demands of the hospital's legal and bureaucratic rules, in addition to whatever is going on in your body.

Soon after you enter the room where you expect to deliver your baby, a nurse takes some blood to make sure your blood is clotting effectively in case you want an epidural pain block. And, since they are sticking you with a needle anyway, they use that same puncture to start the IV. She places a cuff on your arm that inflates every fifteen minutes to check your blood pressure. You also have a little cap on your finger too, a pulse oximeter, that feeds the nurses a reading on your heart rate and the amount of oxygen in your blood.

The anesthesiologist visits you in the birth room. The assumption is that any patient might suddenly need general anesthesia, even though few need it. In order to determine if you can be intubated—meaning have a tube stuck down your throat—the anesthesiologist has you open your mouth wide to check to see if your teeth are loose, has you stick out your tongue to assess how far it extends, and asks you to swivel your head around to ensure you have full neck mobility.

Then they ask you if you want an epidural. First the nurse asks you. Then the anesthesiologist pops by again and says, "When you're ready for your epidural, let me know."

This is a question you are asked frequently, even though you have explained to the staff that you don't want one.

We're talking about the average birth here, so most likely after a time you will be hooked up to the monitor and you will have agreed to an epidural.

Because of the epidural, you are connected to a drip that adds saline to your system so that your blood pressure won't drop dramatically. Attached to your back is the tube to the epidural pump, which feeds a continuous drip of anesthesia into a space around your spinal column. For the average hospital birth, you are hooked up to five machines (blood pressure cuff, electronic fetal monitor, epidural pump, pulse oximeter, and IV) and a catheter has been inserted in your bladder because, with the epidural numbing you, you won't know that you need to pee and you are no longer mobile. Most women on epidurals also end up with Pitocin, a synthetic hormone delivered through an IV drip that accelerates and intensifies your contractions. So at some point after you have entered the birthing room, the nurse will hang a second bag, with Pitocin, on the IV pole.

The arrival at the hospital, with its unfamiliar atmosphere and all the demands of being admitted, plus the epidural slows down your labor. After an initial flurry of noise and activity, the staff leaves you and your birth companion or companions alone, monitoring you remotely from a bank of screens at the nurses' station.

If this is your first child and you didn't hire a doula or a midwife, it gets a little lonely in there trying to figure out what is supposed to happen and if your labor is progressing as it should. The nurse comes in about once an hour to make sure you are not too stressed out, which is not something she can pick up on the screen at the nurses' station and which could stall your labor. Every hour or two, she examines you vaginally to see how dilated you are. If you are not dilating a centimeter every two hours over the course of six or seven hours, they might increase the Pitocin or start saying that your labor has stalled or is failing to progress. If they decide this, you will be getting a C-section, like nearly a third of the women in the hospital.

Before they prep you for the operating room, they suggest a number of things to get labor moving. If your bag of waters, the amniotic sac that surrounds the baby, has not yet broken, a midwife or doctor might suggest nicking it with a device that looks like a crochet hook. This causes a release of prostaglandins and more direct pressure of the baby's head against the cervix, helping the uterus focus the contractions better and speed up the labor. Another technique is stripping the membranes, in which the nurse or midwife or doctor inserts a finger in your vagina and sweeps around under the lip of your cervix to irritate it. This irritation, which hurts, releases a hormone that helps the cervix soften.

When you are fully dilated, the staff tells you it is time to push that baby out. Your epidural is turned down so that you can regain some sensation to push effectively.

After about two hours of pushing, the nurse summons the doctor on call from your doctor's practice. Part of the nurse's job is to alert the doctor of a half-hour window in which the baby will be born so he or she can be there to catch the baby. Your baby isn't coming out as quickly as the doctor thinks she should and the doctor wants to help her along. Although you told your doctor that you don't want him to cut an episiotomy, this doctor is not the one you discussed this with. She grabs a pair of surgical scissors to cut a line from the edge of your vagina toward your anus. She doesn't ask you if you want an episiotomy, and because you are drugged with the epidural, you don't feel the cut until later when the anesthetic wears off.

After your baby is born, the hospital policy is to take the baby to be examined immediately. While the baby is being examined, a nurse gives you a shot of Pitocin to help you push the placenta out. At this point, the active management of your hospital labor is complete.

That term, "active management," is at the heart of the different approaches to giving birth. The hospitals and most doctors approach labor as a crisis. Note how they start you off in the triage, often in a wheelchair too. Are they serious with this triage thing? Triage is a term from the battlefield, an emergency hospital set up so the medical staff can decide which of the wounded can benefit from treatment and who won't survive, a method for allocating scarce resources.

Seems pretty over the top, but it's a window into the medical model of childbirth, the kind that is practiced in most hospitals, the place where 99 percent of women give birth in an atmosphere of crisis. It's a place where pitched battles are fought and American women feel they must come with a defensive birth plan in hand and a small army of supporters to help defend them against the maneuvers of a wily staff who are operating under orders from on high about how birth should be conducted.

What if it didn't have to be this way?

This section will explore the important points you should consider in determining what you believe will be the best birth for you and your child, where you would feel most comfortable, who you want around you, and how you will deal with pain. Most important is not to be afraid. Or at least to face your fears in a way that shrinks them down to a more manageable size and reinforces your confidence about your body and your natural ability to give birth.

Chapter

1

Not Your Mama's Birth Plan

Few first babies arrive on their due dates, Jennifer Jilani had heard, so on the day her baby was scheduled to meet the world, she sent her mom and her mother-in-law, who were visiting for the birth, off on a tourist jaunt to the country and made an appointment for a late afternoon manicure and pedicure. Beautiful toes and fingers for the birth, she thought. The manicurist was brushing the finishing coat of hot pink on her toes when Jenn felt water between her legs. Her water had broken.

She called her husband, Asif, who was working from home, to ask him to join her at the salon and suggested he bring their dog, Senna, who probably could use a walk. Asif was suspicious. Was anything wrong? Had anything happened? Everything was fine, Jenn assured him. She just wanted to walk, and she didn't feel like dragging her bicycle back. Jenn told the manicurist to proceed to paint the fingernails pale pink but not to bother with the cuticles.

This calm and casual attitude about birth was not the way Jenn first approached her birth, but being pregnant in the Netherlands had completely transformed her point of view from the anxiety she naturally felt as an American preparing to give birth. When she discovered she was pregnant, one of her American friends, who had recently had a baby in Amsterdam, referred her to her midwife. "A midwife?" Jenn thought.

"Wasn't that some hippie idea from the sixties?" Jenn told her she wanted to find a real doctor.

Her friend said that in the Netherlands all healthy women see midwives. Only those with dangerous or difficult pregnancies go to doctors. Anyway, Jenn decided, she had to get down to the clinic right away and get checked out. Her friend gave her a phone number for a midwife.

At that first appointment, Jenn was struck by the decidedly unmedical feel of the entire experience. Amsterdam has blocked cars from *De Genestetstraat*, what Jenn refers to as "the birthing block," a street completely devoted to pregnancy and babies. A midwife practice has offices there, along with an acupuncturist who specializes in the discomforts of pregnancy, one of the state-run well child clinics, and a day care center. *De Genestetstraat* also has a children's shop devoted to pregnancy, birth, and babies with a café that caters to moms and offers a special play area for children.

In the midwifery office, instead of chairs lined up stiffly against the walls, there was a big wooden table in the center of the waiting area scattered with information on pregnancy and childbirth, a setup designed to encourage conversation between the couples that gathered around. In brightly colored ink, a mirrored door had a list of the names of the babies the *Het Geboortecentrum* midwives had helped enter the world that week. Facing the street was a big picture window, and women waved to each other as they passed by.

Jenn was charmed, but Asif was alarmed. He called his dad, a pediatrician, to ask him about the Dutch health care system. His father told him that the Dutch system is highly regarded, one of the best in the world. "Maybe I should just allow it to be very low stress," he said. That old familiar stress rushed back when Asif entered the salon and Jenn mouthed to him, "My water broke."

Jenn was grateful she was wearing a long sweater that hid the dampness on her pants. As she and Asif walked, they had to pause when she was overcome by a contraction. When they arrived home, they called their doula, Jennifer Walker (who would provide labor support), and the midwife on call, Mary-Elliz Sheridan, whom Jenn adored.

While Jenn was moving around the living room, sometimes on the couch and other times leaning against the wall to yield to the contractions, Asif was quietly freaking out. He wanted to be at the hospital, which they had decided would be the best thing for a first pregnancy. In the Dutch system, you don't have to decide until the day of the birth where you will have your baby. The midwife calls your first-choice hospital to see if they have a bed available. If not, she continues down the list until she finds an open maternity bed.

Jenn and Asif's moms returned from the tulip fields, and Asif handed them a bottle of wine and two glasses. They set themselves up in the kitchen to wait. Jenn was having heavy back labor. Jennifer Walker used counterpressure and acupressure to help her cope. When Asif came in to the bedroom, he took over digging his thumbs into her hip indentations, while Jenn leaned into the wall. Around 8 p.m., when the contractions were coming faster and harder, the doula suggested that Jenn take a shower and recommended that Asif go in with her to continue to help her.

Around 9 p.m. Jenn entered the bath because Jennifer Walker suggested that probably would help her with the pain. Asif joined her there, holding her from behind as she rode the waves of her contractions. By the time they got out of the tub at around 11 p.m., Jenn had made incredible progress. She was nine centimeters dilated. As Jenn sat in the bath, she had gone through another transition. She realized that she didn't want to go to the hospital. "I couldn't imagine getting dressed, getting in a car," she said. "I couldn't think of how that would separate me from Asif."

When Jenn describes the birth, her mood is light and she focuses on the happy specifics. She remembers the candles Jennifer Walker had placed all around their bedroom and the beautiful soft light they provided. She recalls the mellow and cheerful music of Jack Johnson she had chosen to play in the background. For Asif, as it turned out, the experience was profound.

"I don't think I could have been any more close with her. She was sitting on this birthing stool resting her arms on my legs. I held her arms and rubbed her shoulders. Opposite our bed is a closet with a full-length mirror. We could look each other in the eye. I could see everything. I could see the baby crowning. That was incredible. Quiet and so peaceful and the immediacy of the moment. Jenn gave that last push and immediately the midwife brought our baby to her chest and I could put my arms around them and hold us as a family. Honestly, looking back on it, I could not imagine a better experience," he said. "Within twenty minutes, they had cleaned up the whole place and Jenn and Aleisander and I were in our own bed with our moms at our sides."

The next morning, Jenn's *kraamzorg* (maternity nurse), Grietje, came around 8:30, even though she had been present for the midnight birth. Although Grietje is a private nurse whom the Jilanis hired because they wanted to choose the person, the state pays for a *kraamzorg* to provide care for all moms and babies for two weeks after the birth.

A year later, Jenn's mom, Gail, still cannot get over the beauty of that birth, an event that had her terrified pretty much the entire night. "I have to say it was like going on a journey with her. When she told me she was riding her bicycle at seven months, I wanted to tell her to stop," she said. "Then she was riding that bicycle on her due date! But when I saw her at that birth, it was all so beautiful. My daughter was very, very blessed with everything."

Jennifer Walker agreed with Gail's description of pregnancy as a journey. "You can't have a child without going on a journey, whatever that journey will be," she said. "A woman has to get to know her body, get to know her baby, start to understand her fears, and experience how her hormones change and how what she learns from the people she speaks with along the way affect her ideas about the birth. What she decides at week ten might be the opposite of what she's confident of at week thirty-five. This is a process that puts the woman at the center, and we go on the journey with her. But we don't lead. She does."

Maybe you're hating us right now for describing this beautiful birth story. Oh yeah, you're thinking, everything is beautiful in *the Netherlands*, thousands of miles away from the United States, where the whole friggin' country basically welcomes each new citizen into the world. Just try getting anything like that here. Even if you wanted to give birth like Jenn did, how could you afford it? You might have to pay out-of-pocket for everything!

We present Jenn's story as a way to open your mind to this alternate reality of childbirth, a world where the mother's sense of herself and what she and her baby need drives the process, not the rules of the hospital and the doctor's fear of getting sued. Although this was the Netherlands, you too can have the peace, empowerment, and joy that Jenn experienced even though you are in the United States by doing your homework and assembling the right people around you.

Yes, ours is a system in which we are taught to believe that wisdom and experience reside with the professionals. Our idea of wisdom is a head-centered, brain-focused intelligence that professionals acquire through years of study and training. With that point of view as the starting place, it's difficult to fathom that there is any wisdom residing in the body of someone who has never given birth before. By contrast, in the Netherlands the system is constructed around the wisdom inherent in a woman's body. And yet you can have the best birth for you—despite our system. It's just up to you to advocate for it and by the end of this book, you will know how.

According to a 2008 report released by the Centers for Disease Control (CDC), the U.S. infant mortality rate barely budged between 2000 and 2005, causing the U.S. to slip further behind other developed countries despite spending more on health care. War-torn Bosnia and Croatia have better maternal outcomes than we do. So don't let anyone chide you for being a spoiled, entitled American woman if you go to great lengths to get the kind of birth you want for your family. In fact, you might be saving your life by taking yourself and everyone around you on your journey. This is the first step. Don't look back!

Most pregnant American women do what the Jilanis expected to do: go to their doctors and let the doctors tell them what is going on in their bodies. That's what their mothers did and all of their friends do. After the obstetrician examines her, she goes to the hospital the doctor recommends. Ninety-nine percent of American babies are born in the hospital and only 8 percent of babies are delivered by midwives. It's one-size-fits-all maternity. A woman who wants a birth that reflects her values can arrange for one, but she will have to do her homework.

Unfortunately the burden is on you to arrange all the different circumstances and anticipate the variables as well as think through a plan that clearly describes your preferences. Most women simply walk into the office of the doctor that is covered under their health plan and follow directions from that moment on. Even if that's what you've done, you might consider hiring a doula early on to help guide your journey and accompany you to the hospital. There are always choices!

Sure you can eat right, not drink alcohol, and make sure you do a moderate amount of exercise as a way of believing you have control over your birth. In some ways, that is a bit of control. But the moment you go into the hospital to have your baby, many vital decisions are in the hands of people you've never met. If you want to give birth in a way that reflects your personality and your values, you're going to need to do some homework.

Does that sound like too much of a burden right now? Do you feel like all of this is too much? Geez, can't you just go with the flow and do it the way your mom and your doctor say is the best and the safest? Those are opinions you should consider, but what about your opinion? You know your body and will know your baby better than anyone. You have the power to do this. You can prepare, even though you're not in the Netherlands!

Three basic elements to initially consider when you're pregnant are your body, the baby or babies, and your level of anxiety. Of course, sometimes physical conditions limit the choices of where and how you can have your baby. If you are having more than one baby or if your baby is breech, some midwives will direct you to the hospital and to the care of a physician. For many caregivers, a woman who has a breech baby or is carrying more than one baby is an automatic indication for a C-section. Some midwives and doctors who are experienced in delivering breech babies or multiples vaginally might take you on as a client, but you will have to look hard to find them. Women who have previously delivered children through cesarean section are under a lot of pressure to have their next child through cesarean as well.

Are You High Risk?

A small percentage of pregnancies present dangerous conditions that require the mom to be carefully monitored at the hospital. Like a lot of things related to birth and childbearing, there isn't a uniform consensus on what constitutes a risk. A condition that one doctor might define as high risk might not be seen the same way by a different doctor or a midwife. Many birth professionals don't use the label "high risk" because they see the term as fear-based and subjective.

If a medical professional classifies you as high risk, look further into what these conditions mean, where you fall in the range of risk, and how you might be able to counteract the condition. In some cases, a different care-giver might take a completely different attitude toward your health. In many of these conditions, a midwife can co-manage your care with the help of a physician. Although the pregnancy might need extra monitoring, the delivery of the baby frequently is normal.

The conditions that should concern you are:

Diabetes. If you are diabetic, you have an increased chance of carrying a very large baby, meaning a baby that weighs more than nine pounds, which could complicate labor and delivery. This is also true if you develop diabetes during the course of pregnancy, something called gestational diabetes, a type of diabetes that disappears after the baby is born. Most doctors and midwives treat well-controlled gestational diabetics with diet alone. Some doctors schedule an elective C-section for diabetic women. Some midwives treat the diabetic mom with a carefully managed diet that controls her blood sugar and watch the progress of labor for signs that the baby is too big. It is truly rare for a baby to be too big. We'll address that later in the section entitled "Interventions: The Slippery Slope."

Heart disease. Women with severe heart disease may have trouble with the strain of labor.

(continued)

High blood pressure/preeclampsia/pregnancy-induced hypertension. When a woman has high blood pressure and tests detect protein in her urine, this is a sign of preeclampsia, a very serious condition that can result in seizures while in labor. Preeclampsia can also be defined as elevated blood pressure with severe swelling, or elevated blood pressure with elevated liver function tests or other lab tests (besides simply the urine tests). That's why your blood pressure and urine are checked at every prenatal visit. Hypertension has its own risks to the mom and her baby. High blood pressure in pregnancy carries many complications.

HIV and AIDS. Those who carry HIV or who have AIDS risk transmitting the disease to the baby in the womb, through birth or by breast-feeding. All mothers should be offered screening for HIV/AIDS while pregnant. Transmission of the virus is not inevitable. Careful prenatal care and medications can help decrease the chances of transmission.

Genital herpes. If a woman is suffering an outbreak of genital herpes when she goes into labor, particularly if it is a first outbreak, there is a chance that the baby could contract the virus when coming through the vagina. This poses a serious risk to the baby. If the caregivers determine that the woman is having a herpes outbreak, she will probably need a C-section. If your herpes is not active during labor, question the need for a C-section. In addition, most women with any history of herpes infection are offered prophylactic medication starting at thirty-six weeks to reduce the risk of an outbreak at the onset of labor.

Older age. It used to be that any woman over the age of thirty-five was considered to be high risk because so few women gave birth at that stage in life. With an ever-growing number of women starting their families later— since 1990 there has been a 27 percent increase in women having babies past the age of thirty-five—there has been an increase in the number of healthy babies born to women in this age bracket. If a doctor automatically classifies you as high risk simply because of your age, you probably want to find a doctor who will look at the specifics of your body rather than generally assume that your age equals a risky situation. Midwives care for pregnant women in their forties all the time.

Placenta previa. In rare cases, as the placenta grows it covers all or part of the cervix, a condition known as placenta previa. The placenta may move away from the cervix as pregnancy continues, but if it still obstructs the cervix in the last weeks before labor, doctors plan for a C-section.

VBAC. VBAC, or vaginal birth after cesarean section, is considered to be high risk by some caregivers. A woman's option of VBAC is often defined by the departmental policies of a particular hospital, since, for instance, it must have on-site anesthesia coverage twenty-four hours a day. However, if you are committed to this and are an appropriate candidate, you can seek out the right setting and a caregiver who will assist you in having a vaginal delivery. In some areas of the country, VBAC is disappearing as an option, but it is your right not to be forced to undergo a repeat cesarean. Some women are going to hospitals in neighboring counties or states in order to find a provider who will deliver a VBAC. We'll examine this in much greater detail later in this book.

If you, luckily, don't fit into any of these categories, then you are likely free and clear to pursue the complete spectrum of choices in childbirth.

We'll get into those subjects in greater detail a bit later. For now, let's talk about the worrisome stuff that pretty much every pregnant woman experiences—fear.

Rethinking Fear

For most women pregnancy is a beautiful time filled with happy anticipation and punctuated by stark moments of terror. Feeling yourself fluctuate between these extremes is exhausting. You're picturing the wallpaper of the perfect nursery and swooning over the most adorable little clothes. Just the sounds you make looking through those itty-bitty socks can make you feel like a hormone-stoked fool. The fear isn't that you are shedding so many brain cells standing in the children's clothing department that you might not have enough left to properly care for your child. The discomforting undercurrent is the fear of the unknown and the uncontrollable during childbirth.

Despite your careful preparation, your baby might get stuck some-place in labor, or the pain might become unbearable. Nearly every happy anticipation also presents its opposite. There's the wonderful knowledge that once this baby is born your life will be changed forever. And there's the terrible knowledge that once this baby is born your life will be changed forever. You're vulnerable and dependent. In that state, you have to trust your partner completely. Yikes! When fear spikes, it knocks all those lovely mommy feelings right out of your mind.

There are two sources of fear. There's the externally produced fear you get from talking to other people about their birth experiences and seeing the way television dramatizes birth, and there's the fear you generate on your own.

The way we see birth depicted on television and in the movies is a truly frightening experience. We see none of the softness and peace of the Jilanis' birth. That doesn't make for very good television. The scenes that stay in our minds begin with the maternity ward doors flying apart as the gurney that holds the panicked pregnant woman rushes toward us with doctors and nurses jogging alongside holding an IV bag aloft. Birth in crisis! The disbelieving husband tries to hold his wife's hand, reassuring her that, "It's going to be okay. You're going to be fine. You're doing great." You can see in his eyes that he doesn't believe a word he's saying, and so neither do we. The hero of this scene is not the mom but the doctor. He is saving her and the baby from the perils of her malfunctioning body.

The second kind of fear, the internal kind, takes place within the mysterious inner workings of your body in labor. No matter how many times you hear the elegant choreography of birth described, the hospital scene you've viewed so many times feeds that undercurrent of fear. The horror stories of birth you've heard focus the mind more on what can go wrong than on all the things that usually go right. Yes, labor is a beautiful sequence with one powerful step leading to the next. But each step of the process might stall if your body doesn't work as it is supposed to, and you can't do anything about it.

What they don't tell you is that the first image of birth in some ways prefigures the second. So much of what we think about, yet refuse to really talk about, related to birth in America focuses on fear and the fear of pain. This can influence the stalling of labor, particularly for first-time moms who don't know the rhythm of their bodies in childbirth and, as a result, believe that each pause in the progress of labor is a sign of disaster. And since everyone around them is familiar with the disaster scenario, women have their fears validated by the looks in their companions' eyes.

Fear stalls labor. If you're schooled from the beginning of your pregnancy to focus on fear of all the things that can possibly go wrong, you've got a higher chance of them going wrong at birth. Here is a brief body chemistry lesson to explain how images of scene one affect the internal reality of scene two.

When most other mammals give birth, they retreat to dark, private, protected places where they can labor in peace and safety. (Think of dogs and cats going under the bed to have their litters.) Americans go to the bright lights, bustle, chaos, and strangers of the hospital. We might rationally believe that the hospital is a safe place because, if disaster strikes, there are professionals and equipment to save mom and baby, but our mammalian brain may believe otherwise.

Under stress, mammals produce stress hormones called catecholamines such as adrenaline and cortisol. These are great hormones to have in your system if you need to fight or flee. If a predator comes upon a laboring deer, a surge of these hormones can stop her labor cold and enable her to jump up and get the hell out of there. If you want labor to progress, these hormones are not so good for you.

When they spike, they reroute blood away from the uterus and placenta to the other major organs. This diminishes oxygen to the baby

Babies in the Breech

For most of their time in the womb, babies float freely in the amniotic fluid, flipping around, sticking their little feet and hands out for a stretch as they grow. Sometime around the eighth month gravity and the pressures of the uterus maneuver them into the head-down birth position. Babies at this stage who look like they will present feet first, butt first, or knees first are breech babies; about 3 to 4 percent of all births are breech.

Although midwives and physicians delivered many breech babies successfully for centuries, the common practice for breech babies these days is a cesarean birth, especially if this is a first baby. The American College of Obstetricians and Gynecologists (ACOG) standard is a C-section for breech babies. Generally speaking, the only babies that are delivered vaginally are the ones who are already too advanced in labor for a C-section.

In part this is because many obstetrical schools no longer teach their students how to deliver breech babies vaginally. Midwives who have a lot of experience in delivering breech babies would disagree that a C-section is automatically called for, particularly if a woman has successfully delivered other babies vaginally and has a "tested" pelvis.

There are old and new ways to try to turn your baby into the head-down position. As Abby recalled earlier, when she found out Matteo was breech, she researched moxibustion, a traditional medicine technique in which the practitioner holds a cone of slow-burning herbs, such as moxa or wormwood, as close to your toe as possible without burning you or causing pain. This is a counterirritant, designed to stimulate blood flow and turn the baby around. There is also a chiropractic adjustment used to turn breeches, as well as a procedure involving acupuncture points.

Another technique for turning the baby is version, a method where the practitioner tries to turn the baby by grabbing hold from outside the mother's belly and manually adjusting the baby. A version needs to be done while carefully monitoring the baby for any signs of distress, as there is the possibility that the cord can get caught during the version and create decreased blood flow to the baby as the cord is pinched. Some practitioners feel that attempting a version is a lower-risk procedure than scheduling a cesarean surgery.

Midwife Tricks

Midwives have passed down a number of techniques for turning a breech baby including:

The slanted board. Lie with your feet elevated and your back supported by a slanted board, such as an ironing board, and your head cushioned by pillows. Do this for five to ten minutes, four to five times a day. It should be done on an empty stomach.

The cold treatment. Babies, the midwives say, don't like the cold. They move away from it. Placing a big bag of frozen peas up near the baby's head might encourage him or her to move away from the top of your belly.

Go to the party! Babies, midwives say, like light and music. If you place a flashlight down near the entry to your vagina and play music, your baby might move in that direction. Also, simply talking to the baby might encourage a position shift. "Go to the light! Go to the light!"

Doctors and many others might laugh at these tricks, but they are worth trying—they are unlikely to carry significant risks and they don't cost a dime.

Chiropractors have a trick called the Webster Technique for repositioning the baby. Your midwife should be able to recommend a chiropractor in your area if you don't already have one.

and slows or stops contractions. Catecholamines also inhibit the production of oxytocin, the hormone that stimulates the progress of labor. When they surge, the uterus stiffens and resists contractions. The French obstetrician Michel Odent's research into this showed that the atmosphere of most hospitals stimulates the part of the brain that produces stress hormones. The reason women rely on synthetic oxytocin (Pitocin) given to them at the hospital and fall victim to unnecessary C-sections, according to Odent, is that the lack of privacy and increased stress of a hospital setting inhibit their ability to produce oxytocin on their own.

Most of the time, moms-to-be in the United States are told not to worry about their fears and let the medical establishment handle that part of it. They've got drugs and machines that will save you from agony and uncertainty. Birth is portrayed as an out-of-body experience. However, the way we want to look at it here is through the mind–body connection.

Birth is automatic and involuntary, no matter how much your doctor or the hospital may tell you that it needs to be managed. It is as automatic as digesting your food. You can't control it. If you are not numbed below the waist, you will know when to push without anyone yelling "PUSH!" at you. But fears, expectations, and beliefs can definitely affect its progress. The emotions you experience in labor signal your body, if you are in a safe place, to have a baby, which affects the limbic system, the part of the body that governs the hormones that influence labor.

If you're in a safe place and a calm state of mind, your body will naturally produce the hormones and neurochemicals that help labor progress. The pituitary gland will bathe your system with oxytocin to stimulate contractions, and prostaglandins will pour from the hypothalamus to ripen the cervix.

This is a very big deal, becoming a mom. You've got every reason to be afraid that it won't go as well as you planned or that you or those around you are not up to the task. If you're frightened by your surroundings or by some emotional issue you haven't resolved before labor begins, this onslaught of hormones will stall and so will your labor. That said, what can you do about your fear?

Start to see fear as your friend. This is counterintuitive, of course. Who wants friends they're frightened of? Fear is not the endpoint, but the starting point. What you're frightened of shows you where and how you need to be supported.

The fears are as individual as the women giving birth. Gayle Peterson, a therapist practicing in northern California, has been working on ways to identify and address these fears since the birth of her first child in 1973. She developed a specialty in birth counseling and hypnosis, a four-session model of defining a woman's fears and giving her ways to cope effectively with them.

Your Birth Inventory

When birth counselor Gayle Peterson meets with clients for the first time, she takes them through what she calls "a birth inventory." The following are the fourteen basic questions she asks her clients to help them explore the fears that might stall labor. If you want to go deeper into this area of birth preparation, pick up her book *An Easier Childbirth* or find a birth counselor or doula in your area to help you cope with these issues.

1. Was this a planned pregnancy?
2. What was your initial response when you realized you were pregnant? Have there been any changes in your attitude or feelings since then?
3. How has this pregnancy affected your relationships with your partner and your family members?
4. How will a baby fit into your current lifestyle and plans?
5. Will a baby alter your lifestyle significantly or change your long-term plans? If so, how?
6. What are your impressions and expectations of a newborn?
7. How will you and your partner share responsibilities for the baby during the first year?
8. What do you know about your own birth? What is your impression of your mother's experience of childbirth?
9. If you have given birth previously, what was it like for you? Is there anything you would change if you could? Is there anything you would do similarly the next time you give birth?
10. Do you feel satisfied with your current plans for this child?
11. How do you envision the birth of this baby? What is important to you? Who will be present at the birth?
12. How do you think you will cope with pain during labor? How do you want to prepare for labor?
13. Do you like your body? Do you trust your body's changes during pregnancy and childbirth?
14. Do you have any particular concerns about this baby? About childbirth? About the postpartum period?

Telling a woman that anxiety has an impact on labor but not giving her some way to cope with it only makes her more anxious. These fourteen questions really focus on the way life changes and how you might change once you bring a new member into the family. They are simple questions about practical things. Answered thoughtfully, they can help you explore the places in your relationships that will be tested during and after the birth. Those candid answers can expose the weak spots in the way you have prepared for this child.

By working with those answers, Gayle helps her clients deal with the four or five issues that have the biggest emotional charge and uses counseling and hypnosis to guide them to reframe their attitudes about the things they fear.

For example, if a woman fears she will become just like her mother, whom she doesn't think was a very good parent, Gayle will guide her to focus on the ways she's not like her mom. Or, if she's afraid she'll lose her identity in motherhood, their work will focus on practical things she can do that will shore up her identity once the baby is born.

By addressing those anxieties, Gayle's work shows, labor doesn't have to be a battle. Those who do this exercise honestly battle their fear before labor begins. In this way, the baby can be an opportunity for an incredible amount of growth for you, healing for the family, and getting closer to your partner.

Of course Gayle has tons of examples of this specialty, since she's been practicing for more than thirty years. When we met, she was just back from a final session with a patient who had a frightening recurring dream that she would give birth and the baby would be taken away from her for a long time, then returned to her much older and significantly disconnected from her. In the baby's absence, she was anxious and alone. Gayle suggested she speak to her mother about what had happened at the woman's own birth.

The woman went to visit her mom to discuss this dream and was shocked to find out that she had been taken away from her mother after birth. Her mother sobbed as she recounted her postpartum nervous breakdown for which she had to be hospitalized for six months. This was so shameful for her mother—she felt so guilty about how indifferent she had been to her daughter when they were reunited—that she had kept this secret for more than thirty years. Being able to release the secret at last was cathartic for the woman's mom. When her client related the story to Gayle, she was calm. Her dream made sense to her once this part of her history was explained. She didn't have the dream after that.

If you understand your fears and plan accordingly, you may be able to manage them on your own—without needing certain drugs during childbirth—by using the power of the mind–body connection.

Pain—Take Control of It

The aspect of labor that women seem to focus on the most is how they will handle the pain. Pain is frightening and, thankfully, most of the time we experience it, it comes as a surprise. If you slam your hand in a car door or pick up the handle of a pot without a potholder, you'll jump around swearing and waving that hand in the air to compensate for the searing discomfort. With that as the idea of pain, few would sign up for twenty-four hours of it in labor. Some women who've had epidurals and caregivers who push epidurals often compare using one for childbirth to getting a tooth pulled with an anesthetic, as in, why would you get a tooth pulled without the Novocain? Why would you put yourself through unnecessary discomfort when instead you could just have the shot, relax, and explore the playlists on your iPod?

We believe this is an inept analogy. Don't you think comparing your beautiful little baby to a rotten tooth is just a teensy bit insulting? There is nothing empowering or transformative about having your tooth yanked. Birth equals create. Extract equals discard. The two just don't line up well. Besides, not all women experience childbirth as pain.

Ecstatic Birth

Ina May Gaskin, one of the most respected midwives in the world, says that when she surveyed 151 women, most of whom had given birth at The Farm midwifery center in Tennessee, one-fifth of these women said they had had an orgasm at some point during labor or birth!

So although we're trained to think that childbirth is extremely painful, the truth is that some women do experience orgasm. This is a big revelation, as it hasn't ever been mentioned in a medical text, as far as we know. Even imagining this possibility can take the curse off labor and birth to some extent, since many women have been raised to think that labor pain is some kind of religiously ordained punishment (historically referred to as "the Curse of Eve").

Ina May first started asking women about this because many times it sounded like they were moaning in ecstasy instead of agony. She says that a good labor and birth often sound like the couple is making a baby, rather than having one. So what makes a woman capable of having an orgasmic birth? Ina May said, "It's not so much about an innate capability as that the ecstatic hormones of birth aren't easy to access in the conditions that we now find in most hospitals, with their bright lights and frequent interruptions. To access the hormones that can help create a sense of euphoria, it is necessary to open one's body and to surrender to the powerful sensations of labor, a difficult thing to do unless it is possible to feel absolutely safe and secure. Women who would like to increase their chances of experiencing an orgasmic birth will need to do some research on the subject so that they understand that much will depend upon the choices they make about where and with whom they will give birth."

The kind of woman who's less likely to have it, Ina May said, is "a woman who is afraid she's going to fart."

That needs some explanation.

Ina May and her colleagues developed a principle of birth called the Sphincter Law. (This theory is described in much more detail in her book *Ina May's Guide to Childbirth*.) The basic concept is that the vagina is a sphincter and so are the throat, urethra, and anus. The midwives have observed that when one sphincter opens, all of them do. And part of being completely open is opening yourself to all possibilities, including that of an orgasmic birth.

"You don't need people around who make you feel inhibited," Ina May said. "And being around people who are violators of sphincter law doesn't help."

And she advises that the baby must cooperate too. "I think that it has everything to do with circumstance," Ina May said. "It's much easier if your baby doesn't try to suck both of his fists at the same time because then you have to deal with his elbows. Too many sharp corners would mess up the orgasm."

Okay, I know you're thinking we're nuts right now. If childbirth isn't painful, then why are all these women in labor asking for drugs? What we're saying is that it's not a slamming-your-hand-in-the-car-door kind of pain. The pain escalates and subsides, and there are periods of rest when you can recoup your energy for the next surge of feeling. Caregivers who are trained in ways to help you handle the pain have a number of inventive techniques to minimize the discomfort. The place to start when considering pain is to look at the ways we think or don't think about it.

The Top Ten Non-Narcotic Pain Relievers to Be Used While in Labor

Encouragement. Having people you trust tell you that you're doing great, your baby is doing great, and you're not about to rip your body in half with the next contraction lessens the anxiety you feel, which takes the edge off the pain.

Water. While in the shower or submerged in a tub of hot water, pain subsides for most women. Midwives call it the aquadural. In part this is because anxiety lessens. It's hard to feel tense in soothing water, and in the tub buoyancy also relieves some of the physical pressure.

Birth balls. Make sure that the place where you plan to give birth has a few of those big, brightly colored balls made of strong plastic that you see in

(continued)

the gym. Straddling them spreads out the pressure on your cervix and flopping on top of one can also massage you as you experience another contraction.

Breathing. The old childbirth standby from Lamaze classes is short, rhythmic breaths that allow you to focus on something outside your pain. Another technique is long, slow breaths that release the tension that is building inside you as labor progresses, or fails to progress. HypnoBirthing also teaches specific breathing techniques and self-hypnosis to take you into a relaxed state and create your body's own natural anesthesia.

Acupressure. Experienced caregivers know just what body buttons to push to relieve your pain. They've been trained to seek out and apply pressure to the special spots unique to your body that soothe back labor or ease headaches. If you are planning to give birth without drugs, make sure to pick a caregiver who knows these spots well.

Movement. Walking, dancing, and swaying from side to side all help labor progress and distract you from anticipating the next contraction. Even if you have found a comfortable position, you should move every thirty minutes or so to help shift your baby closer to being born.

Massage. A partner or caregiver who knows how to knead your shoulders and neck can knock you into a lovely state of relaxation that will make the moments between contractions deeply restful and allow you to think about something besides the upcoming sensations. You might want to rehearse this before the big day so your partner knows what soothes you and you don't have to pretend to tolerate a half-assed massage.

Hot packs or cold packs. The numbing effect of cold on the lower back or the soothing effect of a hot compress on the belly, or wherever else needed, works quickly.

Vocalizing. Women are sometimes shy about making too much noise as they labor. Scream out! Lose your inhibitions! Not all of the vocalizing is screaming. Many women deep within the fugue state of labor let out beautiful deep moans that express how their body is adjusting as the baby moves. Whatever the sound you prefer, feel free to make it. Open the mouth, open the cervix, and let that baby out!

Hire a doula. These personal labor assistants are trained to support you emotionally and physically, but not to assist you in the medical aspects of birth as a midwife would. They stay with you for the entire birth and are skilled in all of the above techniques, plus they are a calming, experienced presence at times when your partner or family might not be. Studies say that having a doula can cut labor time in half. Many women prefer the hands-on attention of a doula to having an epidural.

In Ina May's classic *Ina May's Guide to Childbirth* she cites a very interesting study that probed into the way American women think about pain in contrast to the way the rest of the women in the world consider it. In the study, researchers told a group of American women and a group of Dutch women (sorry, we're back to those Dutch women again!) who were about to have their babies in hospitals that pain medication might stall their labor. Two-thirds of the Dutch women gave birth without pain medication while only one-sixth of the Americans did. Two days after their births, when the women were asked about their ideas of pain in childbirth, it was clear that even though both groups of women had gone through the same experience, the American women expected it to be more painful and expected pain relief. They just wanted to be knocked out and didn't really want to think about the effect that would have on the baby. Our cultural schooling in anticipating pain is a big factor in how we perceive the pain of childbirth.

But hey, we're Americans and we're sort of stuck with our cultural expectations. We are trained to think of childbirth as painful, but many women in other countries think of pain as part of the process of giving birth and essentially manageable. This difference in attitude has a huge impact on women's perception of pain. Knowing that these fearful expectations are not universal can make you a little curious though. If it isn't certain that it's going to be unbearably painful, what can you do to manage your expectations in a way that makes the pain bearable? You can't control the pain, only your attitude toward it, as the saying goes. What if you could work on changing that attitude?

Pain—The Impossible Extremes

The automatic response to pain is to say you could do without it. That's not subtle enough, not personal enough for the kind of questions we're raising here. Not everyone has the same expectations when it comes to handling pain. See where you stand on Seattle childbirth educator and doula Penny Simkin's pain scale, below, adapted from her book *The Pain Medication Scale*, co-authored with Ruth Ancheta. Penny has written several very insightful and compassionate books about childbirth as well as a great handbook on labor. Her pain scale is provocative because it allows you to compare your image of the kind of birth you want to a realistic expression of how much pain you feel you can manage. It's a good starting point for discussing with your partner and your caregiver your expectations and tolerances in a concrete way rather than simply saying, "Pain? Do. Not. Want." This scale is a great starting point for discussing with your caregivers how you would cope with labor pain.

+10   I want to be numb, to get anesthesia before labor begins. (An impossible extreme.)

+9   I have great fear of labor pain, and I believe I cannot cope. I have to depend on the staff to take away my pain.

+7   I want anesthesia as soon in labor as the doctor will allow or before labor becomes painful.

+5   I want epidural anesthesia in active labor (4–5 cm). I am willing to try to cope until then, perhaps with some narcotic medications.

+3   I want to use some medication, but as little as possible. I plan to use self-help comfort measures for part of labor.

 0   I have no opinion or preference. I will wait and see. (A rare attitude among pregnant women.)

−3   I would like to avoid pain medications, if I can, but if coping becomes difficult, I'd feel like a "martyr" if I did not get them.

−5   I have a strong desire to avoid pain medications, mainly to avoid the side effects on me, my labor, or my baby. I will accept medications for difficult or long labor.

−7   I have a very strong desire for a natural birth, for personal gratification along with the benefits to my baby and my labor. I will be disappointed if I use medication.

−9   I want medication to be denied by my support team and the staff, even if I beg for it.

−10   I want no medication, even for a cesarean delivery. (An impossible extreme.)

(Adapted from Penny Simkin's Pain Medication Preference Scale © 2001, 2008)

One important point to consider as you rethink labor pain is that it is actually helpful. The spikes of pain help release more oxytocin, a hormone that helps the progress of labor. Plus, coping with the discomfort of the baby moving through you causes you to move and shift the baby into a better position.

Let's assume your baby is facing head down in the uterus, just as he should be, but his head is turned the wrong way for a smooth delivery. He's facing to the side when he should be facing up toward your behind. This pain is hard to handle. The midwife or nurse attending you can coax him to rotate by helping you position your body asymmetrically. One foot up on a chair or one knee on the floor in a lunge will open your pelvis in that direction and give the baby more room to twist around. An experienced caregiver will be able to determine where the baby is in his journey and where he might be caught and guide you to positions that encourage his safe and relatively speedy passage.

Your body is a wonderful guide too. There are some positions that just feel better. Some women report that every contraction is different than the one before and informs their body what position to move into next.

Many women feel great when they spread out over a big birth ball, with the pressure of its forgiving surface relieving the strong sensations and helping to massage the baby down with each contraction. By shifting the body into a more comfortable position, expanding the room for the baby to adjust, the baby wriggles down a bit more, moves a bit closer to being born. With the next contraction, the uterus squeezes in a little tighter, nudging the baby forward. You feel that pain and shift some more. The baby twists a little more and so it goes until you're holding your newborn in your arms.

Some of the doctors we talked to about natural childbirth when we were working on our film dismissed the idea of giving birth without pain medication as a "macho mom" fixation. These doctors inferred that natural childbirth was an elitist experience, a way of separating yourself from the other moms at the playground by claiming bragging rights over those whom you judge as too weak to go all the way. The doctors who said that don't understand that when you tell some mothers that you gave birth without pain killers, they don't envy you. They think you're crazy. Besides, the women who give birth without pain medication would never describe the experience as macho.

"Macho mom is a terrible characterization because it implies pompousness and arrogance and this was the least arrogant thing I've ever done," said Jorie Walker, an Alabama mom who, during the first stage of labor, drove forty-five minutes into Tennessee to give birth to her second baby naturally. She couldn't find a doctor in her small Alabama town who would pledge not to give her an epidural. "Every woman I've ever talked to who has had this experience has a profound humility. It's the experiential equivalent of an archeological dig. I felt powerful and very feminine and connected to all the women who had done this before."

We'll return to fear when we get to the section about putting together your support team, wherein we will deal with fear of your mother. No, we're kidding. Fear of your mother needs its own book. There are fears that come up during labor that are images and expectations from the past that should be dealt with in order for it to go more smoothly; many of them have to do with the people who are closest to you. But first we want to close off this part where we're getting you pumped up to handle this, the birth that is your own creation, by addressing something unexpected, positive, and uplifting while having the additional benefit of being true.

You, The Birth Goddess

Perhaps you don't feel so much like a goddess right now. You're nauseous and cranky and your body is cumbersome. Pregnancy pants with a big elastic front panel do not impress you as being standard-issue goddess wear. Nonetheless, what's happening to you is nothing if not miraculous.

Creating life is goddess work. You are stronger, more powerful, and more focused than you've ever been. Life force is coursing through your body and you are living life in a heightened state of awareness. You are extremely sensitive to smell and taste and to the people, situations, and changes in the atmosphere that might do you or your baby harm. What might make you feel vulnerable also makes you fierce. People better watch out because you will do almost anything to protect your baby.

In this state, you are amazing. You are going to access parts of yourself that you didn't know existed. You are going to face your fears. You have decided to face pain and handle it in a way that makes you most comfortable. Dealing with fear and facing pain are the kinds of things that most people run from as fast as they can, but not you. You are the birth goddess and you will do what needs to be done.

When you come out the other side of this experience, you will be a different woman than when you went in. You will know yourself better and have a much broader sense of what you are capable of doing. You will be smarter and stronger than you've ever been before. Each birth experience is extraordinary, yet at the same time birth is commonplace.

Millions of women do this every year. After the birth of your child, you will be connected to all the women who have given birth across the centuries as well as deeply connected to your baby.

From time to time in this book we will highlight other birth goddesses so you can revel in their extraordinary experiences and perhaps take inspiration from what happened to them and how they handled it. Our first birth goddess is Cindy Crawford. Of course Cindy Crawford is a birth goddess. She was a goddess even before she gave birth. She's Cindy Crawford: beautiful, smart, sexy, funny, and, just like you will be, she was transformed by the amazing way she birthed her babies. Cindy turned her baby around in the womb in one massive act of will!

Birth Goddess: Cindy Crawford

Everybody told Cindy Crawford that the birth of the second baby is supposed to be much easier. After the home birth of her first child, son Presley, Cindy and her husband, Rande Gerber, were able to sit down for a relaxing dinner (albeit on one of those inflatable donuts) only hours later. She believed her daughter's birth would be no problem. Kaia, it turned out, wasn't having any of that.

Kaia was what the midwives call "sunny side up" or posterior—she was coming out face up, facing Cindy's front, which meant that her spine was rubbing up against Cindy's. "With Presley I never screamed out," Cindy recalled. "With my daughter, I was standing on my bed screaming obscenities."

Her contractions never fell into a rhythm during the thirty-three hours Cindy was in labor. Toward the end she was in such pain and so frustrated. Her midwife told her to stand up to give her baby more room to maneuver, but Cindy didn't want to leave her bed and didn't want to stand. She wasn't certain how much longer this labor would go on seeing as she was ten centimeters dilated and still didn't have the urge to push.

Rande got a birth ball and placed it on top of the bed so he could support Cindy as she focused on her next contraction. Cindy stood up and rested on the ball. With the weight off her legs, when the next contraction peaked, she let out a primal sound. As the contraction peaked, she felt her baby rotate inside her into the proper position to be born. "It was a very ET-like alien experience," Cindy said. A few pushes later, Cindy held her daughter in her arms.

Hours afterwards, Cindy was a little disappointed that the second birth hadn't gone as smoothly as the first, a peaceful birth where she had gone inward and meditated. She was surprised at how the second birth had exposed a different side of her personality, a much more raw and not-in-control aspect.

"I don't let myself be that way in life. And so to have this experience that was so unedited in any word or action, that was very liberating as well," she said. "My births both gave me something very different. I learned that's okay and that's a side of me. It makes sense that my daughter's birth was so different from Presley's; I believe that babies come out in a way that reflects who they are."

Chapter

2

Your Best Birth Place

As we mentioned, probably everyone you know who has had a baby has done so in the hospital. We're so focused on what could go wrong that if you tell people you want to give birth anywhere but a hospital, they give you a worried look. Some may suggest that you're endangering your child by taking such a risk. As the birth goddess, you don't have to listen to them. In fact, you don't even have to answer their questions if you think your response might displease them. We know most of us feel compelled to explain and defend our choices. In this chapter we are going to review the upsides and the downsides of each place you might consider having the birth so that you can defend your choice or ignore the skeptics with grace.

To begin with, think about where you will be the most comfortable and secure. Choose a place where you know your preferences will be honored and all decisions will be made with your consent and with the health of you and the baby in mind. You want a place that is flexible in the areas that should give a bit to make you and your family the most comfortable. But you also want competence, vigilance, and tenderness in the areas where swift action might be necessary.

That said, where do you want to be?

There are a few things to consider before making that decision. First let's talk about the hospital since so many births take place there.

In the last thirty years, American women have demanded that hospitals change their ways when it comes to how women give birth. The old standard for birth was the woman isolated in a hospital room and her husband pacing (and smoking) with the other husbands in the waiting room. As women have insisted that other members of their family and friends be present at the birth, hospitals have built special birthing suites that are larger and feature rocking chairs and living room-style furniture to create a more home-like atmosphere. Some even have birthing tubs and big showers in which women can relax and relieve the surges of pain.

Birth Place Choices

The hospital. Most women give birth at the hospital, some of which have birthing suites designed to allow you to give birth and remain in the same room, which has a homey feel and less institutional furniture. Hospitals differ but it's common to give birth in the more clinical-looking labor and delivery rooms and then move to a prettier room for the rest of your stay. Some hospitals offer only standard rooms and birth in the operating theater. If you'd like to labor and deliver in the same room, you will need to seek out a hospital that permits that. So it's a good idea to tour several of the hospitals in your area to see which suits your idea of a good place to give birth.

The hospital birth center. Although facilities vary, most hospital birth centers feature larger-than-average rooms with rocking chairs, Jacuzzi tubs, and the medical equipment discreetly tucked away. They are supposed to feel as much like a home environment as possible. The advantage to these birth centers is that they are in the hospital, so you have quick access to a C-section if necessary and your baby can also be swiftly transferred to the neonatal intensive care unit. The disadvantage, if you're trying for a birth without interventions, is that the hospital birth center still follows hospital protocols

(continued)

strictly. If your labor is not progressing according to the hospital's schedule or the staff has decided that your baby is "too big," you will be transferred out of their birth center.

The freestanding birth center. These privately run facilities cater to women who are trying for natural births and don't want to walk through the hospital doors at all. The rooms are large and there usually is a lounge area and frequently a garden. This means plenty of places to move around in during labor as well as space for your friends and family, if you want them around. Freestanding birth centers don't offer epidurals, but some provide narcotics. Birth center policies differ on this point, so you must ask. If you want stronger pain relief or if intervention becomes necessary, the hospital is often a short distance away. Babies room in and breast-feeding is encouraged.

Home. Birthing your baby at home offers you the most control over the environment and, of course, you do not have to travel at all. The midwives visit you at home for your prenatal exams and the birth. They bring with them medical equipment such as a blood pressure cuff, a Doppler to monitor the baby's heartbeat, and equipment to start an IV. Women who want a water birth often rent a portable birthing tub, and some midwives supply them. Minutes after the baby is born, you will be resting comfortably in your bed with your little one nestled at your side. Statistically speaking, home births have excellent outcomes for mother and baby, though women with serious physical conditions and pregnancy complications are usually advised against them.

A standard part of American pregnancy is the prenatal hospital tour where you and your partner acquaint yourselves with the features of the birthing suite. Everything's upbeat and accommodating on the hospital tour. The tour leader shows you the rooms and their various features and answers your questions in a way that builds your confidence that the hospital and the staff have thought of everything you might need. Unfortunately the tour and the truth frequently don't match up on the big day.

Let's return for a moment to the first birth experience of Jorie

Walker so you'll know why she ended up driving forty-five minutes to Tennessee to have her second baby.

When Jorie was pregnant with her first child, she and her husband toured the local hospital's labor and delivery facility. They were pretty impressed. The tour guide showed them an enormous birthing room, "big enough to hold a huge party, with catered lunch," Jorie remembered. The pregnant women on the tour with her were very knowledgeable about birth and what features they wanted.

Did the suite offer showers? Yes, the guide said, leading the group into a spacious bathroom with a shower that was large enough for two. Did the hospital permit women to use different positions while in labor? Certainly, plus the beds were outfitted with squat bars to help them take these positions safely. The guide explained that the solid-looking detachable bar could fit into holes in the sides of the metal bed posts. Was there a birthing tub to help moms with their pain? Yes, a whirlpool tub, in fact, although they didn't show them the tub on the tour.

Jorie was pleased that everything she imagined she might need for the birth, which she wanted to be free of drugs and intervention, was available at the hospital birth center. She had her birth plan written to that effect and had it approved by the doctors in her practice, including the ones who were on call through her labor and delivery.

The big day came. Jorie and her husband went to the doctor for a prenatal visit and he detected several drops of amniotic fluid on a test strip. He told her that she was having a baby that day and to report to the hospital immediately. Incredulous because there were no other signs of impending labor, she decided to get something to eat first. Like most hospitals, this one prohibited laboring moms from eating or drinking. "To me that was like preparing to run a marathon by starving yourself, but it was hospital policy," she said. When she entered the hospital at 4:30 p.m. they put her in the birthing suite.

By 8 p.m. the nurses' admonitions that she was "not leaving the hospital" until she had a baby convinced her she needed Pitocin, even though the lack of progress was not causing the baby distress of any sort. When the contractions started coming on hard and she wanted to find relief, she asked the nurses to bring her the squat bar. The nurses said they couldn't find it. Hours went by as confusion continued about where the squat bar was. Eventually someone brought it to her.

Jorie asked to use the tub, but the nurse said that "hospital policy" forbade the use of a tub when a woman's water had "broken," even in this instance when only a few drops of amniotic fluid were detected. The tub was in a locked room fifty feet or more from any of the labor/delivery rooms, and no one could remember its ever being used. As it was rarely used, a custodian would have to clean it before anyone could sit in it. Plus there was no way to hook a laboring mom up to the monitoring station at the nurses' desk. The laboring mom would have to get out every hour, wrap herself up, go back to her room to be monitored, and then return to the tub.

Once Jorie got the squat bar, its use was short-lived. The doctor on call insisted that women use stirrups to deliver (a fact that was not discussed when the bar was requested), so the squat bar had to be taken away before the doctor could be called.

From one perspective, this could seem like a comedy of errors, a farce of misdirection. Jorie's group of moms was very well informed and asked good questions when they toured the hospital, but they never realized they had to ask follow-up questions such as if anyone was allowed to use the squat bar or the birthing tub. They basically assumed, as most people would, that if the hospital offered these things, they intended for women to use them.

Jorie laughs about this now but when the features of the hospital that would have aided her natural birth were discouraged and denied by the same staff that said they would support her and her choices, it was much more than an annoyance to her. She was extremely upset, even though the baby was born without complications. When she was pregnant with her second child, she definitely didn't want to return to the hospital. "It was really a typical hospital experience, but it wasn't what I wanted and I didn't want any of my consumer dollars to go to something I didn't want. I couldn't emotionally, spiritually, financially support that again," she said.

Jorie's experience shows how carefully you must question what is really going to be available when you go into labor.

As you walk around the hospital on the tour of the maternity ward or attend an orientation session at a birth center, you need to remember that this is a sales pitch. The people conducting the tour are going to show you all the pleasant features of their establishment. You'll see the most beautiful birthing suite, but the tour most likely will not include the triage room, the grim and clinical first stop when you check in during labor. The birthing suite they show you might have a tub too, or a view of a lovely garden. They'll show you the best room, not the smaller, less well-lit room. If you are in that happy pregnant mood, like Ricki was when she toured the birth center where she gave birth to Milo, in the golden glow of anticipation, all of it can look pretty beautiful.

The style of rooms means far less than the attitudes and behaviors of providers. The hospital's cesarean rate is a better indicator of these than its room décor. Hospitals can use style to co-opt substance.

Great! Maybe it all is beautiful. But you are also a consumer. Deciding where you are going to have your baby is a major purchase; you should go in knowing what you want so you can evaluate intelligently what is on offer. Is privacy important to you? What are your chances of getting a private room after the birth? Maybe you're like Jorie Walker, someone who wants to be able to move around during labor. When you tour the hospital rooms, you can see if there are birth balls and squat bars in the rooms. You can ask how women are monitored. What Jorie needed to ask but did not is if they would let her move around and allow her to be monitored intermittently.

There may be staffing reasons behind the fact that hospital policy requires you to be monitored. In most hospitals, the mother is left alone in her room with her partner for most of the labor. If you know you'll want more personal attention from the staff, it's a good idea to find out what the patient-to-staff ratio is at the hospital and if that ratio remains constant, which may or may not allow you personal attention and intermittent monitoring.

Or if you are frightened that something might go wrong and safety is the main thing motivating your decision, you'll be asking a different set of questions than Jorie did. If your idea of a safe birth is one with minimal management and intervention, then you want to know the percentage of women who have C-sections there. How many have their labor speeded up by Pitocin? How many get epidurals? If you elect to have a C-section, you want to go to the place that does them all the time and to a doctor who is very skilled at the procedure.

Another thing to consider is our widespread assumption that hospital birth is safest because, if there is an emergency, the doctors and the emergency room are standing by to handle the situation. But are they really standing by? Does the hospital have a twenty-four-hour emergency room and an anesthesiologist at the hospital all the time? In smaller hospitals these services are only available during certain hours, which is something you need to establish to feel completely safe. If you needed an emergency C-section at one of these hospitals, who would provide the anesthesia?

Accurate information about the hospital's birth practices and procedures should be readily available, but you'd be surprised by how hard it is to find. There are only two states in the country, New York and Massachusetts, that have a Maternity Information Act, which requires hospitals to publish brochures with their rates of induction, episiotomy, VBAC, and C-section, even though that information is routinely collected by the local departments of public health as required by the Centers for Disease Control. Each hospital has a style, a culture of approved and standard procedures, and it's important to know what those are and that they match up with your idea of a good birth.

For example, in Sleepy Hollow, a town on the Hudson River north of New York City, at Phelps Memorial Hospital Center the C-section rate is 20 percent, a pretty low number when you consider that the national average is close to a third. Thirty miles away at Hackensack University Medical Center in New Jersey, nearly half the mothers get C-sections. Phelps has midwives on staff and an acupuncturist who specializes in pregnancy and labor. The hospital also features a birthing tub. If you were touring Phelps, they would be sure to mention these features to you and it would be another sign that you were in a hospital that supports delivery choices and pain relief options that are outside the norm.

Also, the C-section rate within an individual practice can be more telling than the hospital's rate. A hospital can include one group of doctors with an extremely high C-section rate as well as a midwife group with a rate that is much lower. Even though both groups can have access to a Jacuzzi and birth balls, they may not make use of these at an equal rate.

Birth Goddess: Kathy Herron

One determined person can change the culture of birth at a hospital and Kathy Herron is proof of that.

When Kathy Herron first started working at Phelps Memorial Hospital in New York's Hudson River Valley, the staff thought she had magic hands. Kathy had been delivering babies with a population of mothers on Medicaid through a midwifery practice for about a decade, most of which had been natural deliveries. When the hospital she had been working with closed down, she showed up at Phelps. "They were like, okay, what's a midwife?" Kathy remembers.

During the first delivery she supervised, she got lucky in terms of making a good first impression. "It was a very normal delivery. I just caught the baby as she came out of the mom," Kathy said. "For two weeks people just came up to me and asked if it was true. She didn't have an episiotomy? She didn't have her legs in stirrups? She didn't have an IV or any kind of medication? I had been in other hospitals where this sort of thing was unusual but this was an extreme reaction."

By the second birth, the staff was really paying attention. The mom Kathy was working with was pretty far along in labor, sitting in a rocking chair in the birthing suite. The attending nurse told Kathy that she had to get her back in the bed and get her feet into the stirrups. Kathy said that would be too much for the mom at this stage. Kathy quietly asked the nurse to bring over the supplies and the baby fell right out into Kathy's hands.

When she looked over at the nurse, she was standing there with her mouth open, tears in her eyes.

Suddenly many nurses were saying, "Let's not put her feet in stirrups. That's not how Kathy does it."

(continued)

Doctors came to watch Kathy deliver babies. Some of them were not persuaded and others were intrigued. "But pretty much all of them were plastered up against the wall when the mom was delivering," Kathy said. "They'd ask me if it was true that I never cut episiotomies for first-time moms. I said I didn't think it was really necessary."

Years later, after she had established her credibility with the administration, she decided to start a private practice and asked to have delivery privileges at the hospital. The head of the obstetrics department surprised her by saying that the hospital would love to have her. This means that she and her partner are the only midwives who are not employees of a doctor and who have admitting privileges at any hospital in Westchester County.

Phelps has welcomed two additional practices with midwives and now boasts the lowest C-section rate in the county. Kathy is using her credibility to lobby for more unconventional maternity services such as birthing tubs. She persuaded the hospital to install one over the objections of some members of the medical staff, who thought no one would use it. "Now women are fighting over it," Kathy said. "Slowly and steadily."

The following is a list of questions you should ask the hospital when you are trying to decide where to have your baby. When we were writing up the list we thought, "Wow, this is really long. Aren't people going to feel like a total pain in the ass going down to the hospital with this list and interrogating the staff?"

But, as Jorie Walker's experience shows, it all fits together, with one thing definitely influencing whether you can get another. For example, in many hospitals it is standard to hook a laboring mom up to an IV right after she has been admitted in case she needs emergency fluids or quick access to a drug. Once the IV is in, she can't walk around as easily or use the shower or the tub for pain relief. If the protocols allow for a Hep-Lock, which is a portal into your vein that is not yet attached to an IV pole, you can move around, get in the water, and still be available for emergency hookup to the IV. So what seems like a small difference could make a big difference in your choices in labor.

If you've done all the work of visualizing an ideal birth, psyching yourself up for a particular kind of pain relief, thinking that you and your partner will be a fabulous team, then you do not want to be surprised by some arcane hospital rule that interferes with this intimate experience. How many times have we heard of couples who have come to the hospital happily toting their video cameras to film the birth only to be told that the hospital rules don't allow that? They might not want you to have a visual record in case something happens during the birth that results in a malpractice suit.

Or women who have depended on the support of a doula with whom they've built a vital bond, only to find that the hospital only allows one person, a family member, to attend births. So even though this list of questions we've developed looks awfully long and overly detailed, not a single one of these questions is irrelevant, as far as we're concerned. You can pick and choose which matter to you depending on how you envision your best birth.

Questions for the Hospital Tour

These questions cover a wide range of birth choices, some of which might be irrelevant to the way you want to give birth. Maybe you don't care if there's a birthing tub. Maybe you don't really mind being hooked up to a monitor. Just ask the questions that are important to you.

- When should I come to the hospital?
- When will the nursing staff tell my caregiver to arrive?
- What non-drug pain relief is available? A squat bar? A shower? A tub? Are these routinely used by laboring women?
- Are you open to natural methods of pain management and birth, to water birth or HypnoBirth?
- Will I be allowed to move around?
- Is continuous monitoring standard?
- What is the rate of IV use? Is a Hep-Lock available instead?

(continued)

- Can I stay in one room or will I be moved from room to room as my labor progresses?
- What are my chances of getting a private room after my baby is born? Is there a special procedure to request one?
- Do you honor birth plans? To whom should I give my plan? Who do I speak with if I think that my plan is being ignored?
- How often do you augment labor? How many mothers are put on Pitocin?
- What percentage of moms get epidurals?
- What is your C-section rate? Your VBAC (vaginal birth after a cesarean) percentage?
- Do you allow doulas to attend births?
- Will I have unrestricted access to my partner and my birth companions?
- If I need pain relief, who do I ask?
- What is the patient-to-staff ratio? Is that ratio consistent twenty-four hours a day?
- What if I am not getting along with my nurse? Can I ask for her to be replaced? What is the procedure for that?
- Is this a teaching hospital? Will medical students and trainees be giving me vaginal exams and other procedures?
- Can I wear my own clothing?
- Do you allow videotaping of the birth?
- Will I be allowed to eat and drink during labor?
- What is the hospital's emergency capability? Do you have a twenty-four-hour emergency staff and an anesthesiologist present at all times?
- What is the policy immediately after birth? Can I hold my baby right away? Or will you be testing and examining her?
- Does the hospital allow newborns to stay with their mothers, rooming in?
- Can I have the baby stay with me after the initial examination and not be taken to the nursery right after birth?

You've got to be savvy in the way you ask your questions. Maybe you find out you can wear your nightgown and your partner can be with you all the time but the only doulas they allow are ones that are known by the doctors and hospital staff. That might be an indication that either you need to find a doula who works regularly at this hospital or, if you like the doula more than the hospital, find a different hospital.

If you ask them if you can move around, they'll probably say yes. You also need to ask if the hospital mandates traditional IVs because once that is attached to you, you may not be able to move anymore or they may allow you to push the IV pole as you walk around.

Positions for Childbirth—They're Not What You Think

In the United States, when we envision a woman in labor, we picture her lying down on her back in bed with her feet in stirrups. That's what you'd find in most hospitals here, anyway. The truth is that this position may not be the best one for normal childbirth. If you're lying on your back, you're not allowing gravity to play a role that can actually help the baby move down the birth canal.

In *Ina May's Guide to Childbirth*, Ina May discusses the importance of being able to change position and move freely. She says that in the first stage of labor, this helps dilate the cervix and bring the baby into a better position to pass through the pelvis. She suggests sitting on your partner's lap, a birthing stool, a birth ball, or even the toilet if you can (of course, this means that your movement can't be hampered by an IV, an electronic fetal monitor, or an epidural anesthesia).

Elsewhere in the world, women commonly labor while sitting, kneeling, standing, slowly walking or swaying, squatting, lying on her side, or in a hands-and-knees position—or various combinations of these. These positions can help with pain relief, and they can help to continue moving the baby down the birth canal. If you're curious, talk to your caregiver about trying these positions, particularly since the possibilities will be dependent on

(continued)

the other interventions you have, the size and position of the baby, and the progression and stage of your labor. Keep in mind that some hospitals will actually allow for these positions, despite what you may assume. If you feel strongly about trying different positions, be sure to let your birth team in on this so they can advocate for you if necessary. You are not going to want a nurse to come into the room and try to get you to lie down on your back in the middle of a contraction!

Don't ask, "May I refuse an epidural?" Of course you can refuse one, but will the staff keep pressuring you until you finally give in? Instead, ask what percentage of mothers giving birth in this hospital have epidurals. In some hospitals that figure can go as high as 90 percent. If that figure is the answer, you know that you'd be under considerable pressure to conform to the hospital's expectations. In labor you might not be in the best condition to resist that momentum. This would be a strong indication that you should look at other hospitals or instruct your birth team to support you vigorously in resisting the pressures of the staff.

If, when asking these questions, you find it's difficult to get the answers you want or the staff gives you a lot of attitude, you might want to look elsewhere. You don't want to be giving birth in an environment that feels like enemy territory. When you are in labor in a hospital, you will be relying on the hospital and the staff. Even if you love your obstetrician, he or she may not be with you until the final stage of pushing.

Certainly hospital maternity wards have made a lot of progress in accommodating the wishes of moms in the last thirty years. They can always do more, however, and they won't be inclined to do so unless consumers show them that these attitudes and practices are unprofitable. Only by women asking questions and demanding changes will hospitals begin to change their ways. Birth is big business for these hospitals and they should go out of their way to make you comfortable and to assure that they run the kind of operation whose idea of a good birth matches yours. That's a place where you'll have an increased chance of getting the kind of birth you want.

The Birth Center

If you think the hospital is too medicalized and clinical, the middle option is a birth center. Some hospitals have birth centers attached or even inside the building, like the one where Ricki had Milo. There are also free-standing birth centers (typically close to a hospital) run by midwives or financed and operated by a combination of midwives and doctors.

Their primary purpose is to create a safe place for women to give birth that has a strong connection to the medical establishment for those who are not comfortable having their babies at home. The idea is not to be a mini-hospital, but rather to be a maxi-home, a place with a homey feel but with an affiliation to a hospital in case intervention is necessary.

The difference between freestanding birth centers and the ones attached to the hospital is that hospital birth centers follow hospital rules. The midwives are able to give you more flexibility but they still have to adhere to the hospital policy. As a birth center, it's got a homey feel and the birthing suites have better furniture. We don't want to mislead you into thinking, when we say "birthing suite," that you're going to be having your baby in the penthouse of the Four Seasons. Like we said about the hospital-based birth center where Ricki had Milo, it's not exactly decorator décor. You'll have a double bed and a bit more freedom to move, but it's still the hospital, and you're on the hospital timetable and must follow the hospital protocols. Some women like this melding of styles because it offers access to all of modern medicine but with the look and feel of home (or as close as you can get to that while you're still close to an operating room).

If you decide midway through the birth that you would benefit from an epidural or labor augmentation, you can often transfer seamlessly into the standard labor and delivery area. You also have quick access to a C-section if necessary and your baby has access to pediatric emergency care. Hospital birth centers typically have a nursery, although they encourage babies to room in.

Don't be misled by hospitals that market their labor and delivery ward as a "birth center" or their rooms as "birthing suites." A true hospital-based birth center is staffed by midwives and other professionals who are experienced in supporting natural deliveries. It is in a separate wing, floor, or building from the hospital's labor and delivery ward, which is staffed by residents. Some OB-GYNs will attend deliveries in a hospital birth center, but anesthesiologists do not, so there is no option for epidurals.

The freestanding birth center is an independent business venture run by midwives or a medical practice that hires midwives. There are big, bustling birth centers with large staffs of midwives that can handle forty births a month, and much smaller operations that can only take on a maximum of ten or fifteen. What different birth centers offer can be as varied as the people who operate them all, with a common goal of more personal care.

What's the Deal with Water Birth?

Although women have given birth in water for centuries worldwide, water births didn't start to become more popular in the United States until the 1980s. It is now often used in conjunction with other natural methods such as the Lamaze and Bradley birthing techniques.

Women are drawn to water birth for the benefits it offers them and the baby. For you, the warm water promotes relaxation, helps labor progress, makes it easier for you to move around comfortably because you're weightless, and relieves pain by taking pressure off the uterus. Water softens the perineum (the area between the anus and vagina), making it more pliable, which helps ease the birth.

For your baby, transitioning from the amniotic fluid to warm water to the air is a less shocking way of entering the world. Some say that this is a "kinder" method of birth for the baby.

A water birth doesn't automatically mean you won't have access to IV medications while you're in labor (ask your caregiver for more information if you think you want access to certain drugs but are still interested in a water birth).

Some women like to have the birthing tub available nearby while they labor, choosing to get in only when they are about to birth the baby. Others choose to labor in water and then get out of the tub for delivery.

Some hospitals now offer birthing tubs, and many birth centers include them as well (if you're interested, ask during the tour). Of course, if you choose to birth at home, water birth is an option—either in your own bathtub or in a portable birthing tub that your midwife may provide. Not all midwives are trained in water birth, though, so make sure this is a conversation you have early on if you feel strongly about having water birth as an option.

Women who have their babies at a freestanding birth center usually have had a good portion of their prenatal care there and have taken childbirth preparation classes with the staff. These centers also typically offer well-woman care and lactation support. By the time the baby is about to be born, both mom and partner are well-acquainted with the staff. The atmosphere is emotionally supportive. There is no admission procedure. Your records are already there when you arrive for the birth, so you don't need to fill out a stack of papers, and there's nothing for you to sign. There are no visiting hours or restrictions on who is with you.

One nice feature of freestanding birth centers is that they usually have a common room with big comfy couches that lend it the feeling of a living room. This allows a woman in labor more places to roam when she's trying to find comfortable positions to help her labor progress. Friends and family can be near, but there is also space for privacy when the couple wants time alone. If you'd like your family and friends to be around, they can hang out in the common area. In many cases, birth centers also have a garden or a patio and a kitchen so your supporters can make you the kind of food you like. Freestanding birth centers typically don't have a nursery. Hospital birth centers do, although they also encourage babies rooming in. Stays in a birth center are generally short, often twenty-four hours or less.

In many ways, the advantages of a freestanding birth center are similar to those you have at a home birth. Centers are staffed by nurse midwives, certified professional midwives, and trained birth attendants. They have oxygen on hand and can start IVs if needed, just like midwives at a home birth. Those that are licensed by the state are capable of handling many emergencies. Additionally, centers that are accredited by the American Association of Birth Centers, a lengthy, expensive, and rigorous process, do not insist on continuous fetal monitoring, only intermittent. Some centers offer narcotic pain relief such as Demerol, morphine, or Stadol, but they cannot provide epidurals. They also can administer Pitocin, if needed, to help the mom deliver the placenta after the baby is born, or to control postpartum bleeding.

A big advantage of freestanding birth centers is that the best ones have a long established relationship with a hospital nearby, where the midwives may have privileges and are well known by emergency personnel. They are usually just a few minutes from a hospital for a quick transfer if the birth gets dangerous or too painful for the mom to bear. If the midwives have privileges there, they often are allowed to stay with you throughout labor in the hospital and advocate for your care there. Also, freestanding birth centers may be able to accommodate VBACs and offer water births, which hospital-based birth centers typically do not. If you have a VBAC attended by midwives, you will generally not be able to deliver in the birth center and the hospital will require you to have continuous fetal monitoring.

All birth centers have much lower C-section rates than hospitals. The national average for birth centers is about 4.5 percent. Nearly 16 percent of those who start off their birth at a birth center transfer to the hospital and about a third of those are for C-sections. The other two-thirds usually transfer because the moms or the midwives decide an epidural is needed.

What to Look for in a Birth Center

You want a center that is clean, well organized, and professional. During the orientation, the center should have handouts describing the services it offers and, if it's a freestanding birth center, what hospital it is affiliated with.

The staff should tell you if there are certain types of patients they do not serve, such as if they have restrictions on the weight of babies they will deliver or if they cannot handle you if you need to be induced. All of this information should be available to you during the orientation to help you decide if you and the center are a fit. Other questions you want to ask include:

- Is the birth center licensed by the state? (The answer must be yes.)
- Is it accredited by the American Association of Birth Centers Commission for the Accreditation of Birth Centers? (The answer must be yes.)
- Is there a library at the birth center where I can borrow books, CDs, and DVDs on pregnancy and childbirth?
- Are the handouts thoughtfully put together? Do they look professional?
- Does the center take my insurance? If not, what kind of insurance does it accept?
- Who is the consulting physician for the birth center, and when will I get to meet him or her?
- Where is the backup hospital?
- Do the birth center providers have hospital privileges?
- Are all the members of the staff trained in infant resuscitation? (The answer must be yes.)
- How many women are transferred to a hospital while in labor? Before labor? After the birth of the baby? Can the members of the birth center staff stay with the mother in labor and delivery if they do not have hospital privileges?
- What are the most frequent reasons for a hospital transfer?
- How will the center help me manage pain?
- What is the rate of episiotomies? How often do moms have their bag of waters ruptured and under what circumstances?

(continued)

- What methods do midwives at this center use to get labor to progress?
- Generally, at what point in labor does the staff recommend I come to the birth center?
- Can I hire my own doula?
- Are there restrictions that could prevent me from using the birth center? Are there limits on the size my baby can be? Do you limit the length of labor or bar women whose pregnancies go past forty-one weeks?
- Does the center do vaginal births after a C-section (VBAC)?

Many women go through a point in labor, as Ricki did during her home birth of Owen, when they think they just can't take the pain anymore and the whole thing is going on too long. This is called the transition phase, when a woman is typically dilated eight to ten centimeters, contractions are stronger and more frequent (every few minutes), and she typically feels an overwhelming urge to push. If she can get through that moment, things typically commence fairly quickly toward delivering the baby. If a mom laboring in a birth center wants an epidural, she must transfer to the hospital to get it. Having to get up, change clothes, get in the car, and be admitted to the hospital is a big drama. Because of that, many moms decide to tough it out and go through with a drug-free birth. So if you'd like the option of getting an epidural, a freestanding birth center may not be the right choice for you.

Currently there are only 175 birth centers in the whole country. The economics of birth are daunting for these private operations and recently two birth centers we were familiar with in New York City closed down. When we were trying to find one in Los Angeles early in 2008, we discovered with sadness that one that had been operating for nearly a decade had recently closed. The closest one available to the thousands of women who get pregnant every year in Los Angeles was in the next county north of L.A. So before you decide a birth center is the ideal middle ground that solves the problem of your fear of hospitals and your fear of giving birth at home, you need to find out if there is a birth center near you that is accredited by the American Association of Birth Centers.

If there is no birth center reasonably close to where you live, Kate Bauer, the executive director of the American Association of Birth Centers, recommends that you write to her association (see the resources section at the back of this book for the address) and request a brochure on what birth centers offer. Armed with this brochure, go to your local hospital and discuss with the staff the elements of birthing at a birth center that you wish they offered in their maternity ward. Working with a midwife in a hospital or at home can be a great solution if there are no birth centers near you. The only way for all women to be able to choose what the birth centers offer is for consumers to start asking for it.

Birth Centers Closing

The golden age for birth centers was the 1980s when a combination of factors caused them to spring up around the country. Certified nurse midwives wanted a place where they could practice the midwifery model of care without interference by doctors. As natural childbirth was becoming better established, women were seeking out alternative ways to give birth. When Jan Lobatz and her midwife partners opened the Maternity Center in Bethesda, Maryland, in 1982, they had a steady number of customers right from the start.

They felt like they were breaking new ground in other ways. They were extremely grateful to the kind and compassionate doctors who provided the medical backup required by the state, but they also liked the shift in the power dynamic. "We liked the idea of midwives paying doctors instead of the other way around."

The practice flourished, requiring the Maternity Center to keep expanding.

Then the insurance companies ruined the business.

The combination of shrinking reimbursement for births from the insurance companies and skyrocketing malpractice fees squeezed Lobatz to the point where it was impossible to keep the doors of the birth center open.

Lobatz had to cut back staff as the number of clients started to decline. There were still customers desiring the service, but the business was operating

(continued)

on such a thin margin that even a small decrease was difficult to absorb. Gradually it got to the point where neither she nor any of her partners had a very good quality of life. "It seemed like I was always on call and we couldn't pay the staff the kind of benefits we wanted to pay them," Lobatz said. "Then it got to the point where I couldn't pay my bills."

Kate Bauer, the executive director of the American Association of Birth Centers, acknowledged that just like in any other small business, new birth centers open and some birth centers close every year. Generally, centers that close in the first few years of operation do so because they are undercapitalized. An AABC survey of closed centers found that those owned by hospitals or physicians are more likely to close. Nonprofit community birth centers or those owned by midwives tend to have greater longevity. The boards and owners of these centers are passionate about the care they provide and resourceful when challenges present themselves. A new trend is that some birth centers are branching out to retail, opening organic baby boutiques or vitamin shops to offset ever-increasing operating costs.

Carol Leonard, the first certified professional midwife in the state of New Hampshire, almost had to close down her birth center in 2003 because no private insurance companies would reimburse her for services. At the time, she was charging $4,000 per birth and the local hospital was charging approximately $13,000. She met with several insurers to figure out why they wouldn't reimburse an option that is cheaper and statistically safer. The insurers told her that not enough women want this "option" to justify the cost–risk analysis they would need to do in order to cover it. Eventually Leonard prevailed and was able to convince the insurance companies to cover her services. Recently, New Hampshire passed a state law mandating that all insurance companies cover the costs of a home birth.

There was a tremendous outcry in the community when the Maternity Center announced it was going to close. Women who had had their children at the center back in the eighties were looking forward to their daughters' giving birth there. It was hard on Lobatz too. Of closing her center in 2007, Lobatz said, "I was very, very traumatized by the closing of the birth center. It was my baby. But it's a business and you have to run it like a business."

The issue of insurance reimbursement is something to consider if you want to use a freestanding birth center. Birth centers negotiate contracts for reimbursement with some insurance companies. Check with the staff of the birth center to see if it is under contract with your insurance and if the payment process for the birth center will be similar to that with a hospital. Similarly, if you want to use a hospital birth center, check with the staff to make sure that they take the same insurance as the hospital itself.

If the center has no contract with your insurance carrier, the insurance company typically only pays a portion of the birth center's fee, usually half. You'll be required to pay the difference. Judi Tinkelenberg, who runs Community Childbearing Institute in San Francisco, requires patients whose insurance doesn't cover the full cost of birth to pay in full before the birth. She said once the baby is born, it was nearly impossible to get the final payment from the family, who suddenly had other ways it wanted to spend its money.

Home Birth

Home birth in America is growing in popularity but still very rare, which is too bad when you understand how sweet and safe it can be for a normal pregnancy. You can have your baby in your own bed with your partner and your family right there beside you. Along with them, you can have a clinically skilled midwife deliver your baby. She's also someone who is alert to the signs when something is going wrong, and is trained to deal with complications.

The advantages of being cared for by a home birth midwife take place throughout the pregnancy, not just on the day of the birth. Prenatal care is typically conducted during visits at home and the appointments are lengthy and personal. There is plenty of time to talk about what is bothering you physically and emotionally about the upcoming birth and to develop a strong relationship with the woman who will be attending you.

But it's not all hand holding and here's a box of tissues. Since midwives are medically trained, she can help you decide about sonograms, amniocentesis, and other high-tech testing you and she decide might be appropriate. A few midwives even offer the option of a fetal heart rate monitor for the birth, if that's what would make a mom feel more comfortable.

Home birth midwives carry oxygen, Pitocin, and Methergine (medication to control hemorrhages) and are extremely well-trained in infant resuscitation. If you test positive for group B strep (10 to 20 percent of pregnant women test positive for this common bacteria that lives in the vagina and can be harmful to newborns), they can administer the same antibiotics you would receive in the hospital. They bring anesthetic and equipment for suturing vaginal tears and can withdraw umbilical-cord blood for cord-blood banking. They will perform all the routine newborn tests and give the baby any medications that are state-mandated. They also guide you through the process of applying for a birth certificate.

Despite the rigorous professional training and strong experience of midwives, if you tell your family this is what you are planning, they'll probably think you've lost your mind. When Jill Williams told her family that she wanted to have a home birth for her third child, they didn't want her to do it. "I told my mother via e-mail and then she didn't answer the phone for a while," Jill said. "We didn't tell people we were doing home birth after that because we didn't want to hear the reaction. People would say we were crazy or 'better you than me.' One person in the supermarket told us we were endangering our baby. 'Don't you value your baby's life?' she asked. After that we just stopped telling people what we wanted to do."

Jill had come to believe that a home birth might be safer than one in the hospital after what she'd been through. Her first child was induced unnecessarily, Jill believes, when she was only six days past her due date. The Pitocin gave her blockbuster contractions and her nine pound, nine ounce baby made a huge tear in her vagina. She thought this wouldn't have happened if she'd been allowed to deliver naturally, as she had wanted to do.

For her second child, she had a small placenta previa, meaning a piece of the placenta covered the opening to the cervix. At thirty-four weeks the problem resolved itself, but she felt it was too late to arrange for a home birth. The doctor recommended she schedule a C-section because of the placenta previa, even though it was no longer a problem. Jill stayed at home until she was nine centimeters dilated before she headed to the hospital so that she wouldn't be drawn into the C-section plan.

At first she and her husband wanted to take the middle option of a birth center for their third child, but there were none near their home in Lexington, Kentucky. After the experiences they'd had at the hospital, they were adamant that they wanted this one at home. They found a certified nurse midwife, Donna Galati, who was willing to attend the birth.

The night she went into labor, Jill and her husband went to dinner, put their daughters to bed, and waited for Donna to arrive. When she showed up it was around 8:30 at night. Donna found that Jill was at nine centimeters. "I wanted to have my baby by midnight," Jill said. "I asked her to break the bag of waters (tear a hole in the amniotic sac) and get this thing going."

When Donna complied, the pace quickened. Knowing that the baby would probably be big because Jill's other children had been quite large, Donna used oil to massage Jill's perineum, the tissue between the vagina and the anus, to keep it supple. "The pushing was hard, probably the hardest work I've ever done, but I only had to push for forty minutes," Jill said. The reason that Jill had to work so hard was that her baby was over ten pounds. So big, Donna said, that they weighed her on two different scales to convince themselves this was so.

We're talking about a petite woman who delivered a baby that was over ten pounds vaginally at home without a drop of medication, intervention, or cutting.

One enormous factor in this smooth birth was that this was not Jill's first baby. Still, what she liked, and what most home birth moms like, is the fact that, well, it takes place at home. The atmosphere is not full of rushing and frenzy as if a disaster has just befallen the family. Jill's girls were sleeping in the next room and woke up to greet their new sister.

Nonetheless, home birth is not for everyone. Many women feel this kind of birth is risky, as Jill's parents did. Having your baby at home is legal in every state in the United States, but using a particular type of midwife may not be. Therefore you may have to travel to a neighboring state where you can find a licensed midwife. All the women interviewed for this book who have had successful home births said they definitely want to do it the same way for their next child. This is not the overwhelming conclusion of women who have given birth in the hospital.

There are some midwives who can offer you the choice of a home or hospital delivery. For example, Amy Willen and her partner Jennifer Gagnon are two of three nurse-midwives in Chicago who attend home births and have hospital privileges. Their practice offers the same options that women receive in the UK, where they can choose at any point during the pregnancy or labor whether they'd prefer to be at home or in the hospital.

Amy knows firsthand that there is a lot of demand for this service. "We turn away people every week, at least three a week," she says. Amy and Jennifer love the autonomy they have to serve women in the way they think is best. "We don't have to answer to a hospital administrator with regard to the number of patients per hour that we see, or to an MD employer that holds us to MD productivity standards," said Jennifer. "We can schedule thirty- and sixty-minute-long appointments."

The option of being able to deliver at home or in the hospital with your midwife and not have to transfer into the care of an obstetrician is very appealing. But for reasons we will explain in the midwives chapter, it can be challenging for a nurse-midwife who attends home births to obtain hospital privileges or collaborations with physicians due to the negative bias against home birth in the medical community.

Nearly every woman in America gives birth in the hospital, but when women in Sweden and England were randomly assigned to birth their babies in either birth centers or hospitals, 80 percent of the Swedish women and 75 percent of the British women who were assigned to the birth centers gave the centers their highest satisfaction rating. Only half of the women who were randomly assigned to a hospital birth said they wanted to return there for their next baby.

Is Home Birth for You?

A home birth can be a beautiful event, but it's not for everyone. Women who choose home birth believe it is safer. They do not run the risk of unwanted hospital interventions and birth takes place in an atmosphere they control. In birth, however, not everything is completely under your control. If the idea of a home birth appeals to you, here are a few things to consider before committing:

- If you are high risk (see "Are You High Risk?", p. 13), a home birth is not for you.
- Consider the distance to the hospital, especially if you live in an area that can have a lot of traffic or is so remote that you're more than thirty minutes from the nearest hospital.
- What will your plan be if your pregnancy becomes difficult with bleeding, high blood pressure, or premature labor?
- If you are having twins, a breech birth, or a vaginal birth after a C-section, some home birth midwives prefer you to be hospitalized. Some are comfortable assisting in these births, however. Ask.
- Consider if you are unsettled about your capacity to handle the pain of labor.
- Consider if you are having a lot of anxiety about the birth.
- How will you proceed if you can't find a qualified attendant who will commit to your home birth?
- What will be your plan if your insurance doesn't cover home birth or is unclear if it will? Some states mandate reimbursement for home birth from insurance companies, while others allow the insurance companies to determine what to cover. Your midwife will be very familiar with the insurance situation in your area, and many of them have become quite clever in getting full or partial reimbursement.
- Will you be comfortable at home? Do you have enough privacy, space, or support?
- How will you feel if you are not certain that your partner will support you fully?

The obstetricians' professional society (ACOG) opposes home birth, regarding it as very dangerous to mother and baby and dismissing those who want to have their babies at home as falling victim to what is "fashionable, trendy, or the latest cause célèbre." In fact, in May 2008 the American Medical Association (AMA) issued a resolution against home birth that singled out Ricki for sharing her experience on the *Today* show and in our documentary. Stressing their one-sided view, they warned that a normal delivery can become complicated very quickly and the safest place to have a baby is in a hospital or a freestanding birth center that meets their standards. The resolution instructed the AMA staff to create model legislation that would claim hospitals or birth centers as the safest places to have a baby.

Not everyone agrees with this, though. In a recent statement, the National Perinatal Association supported home births for low-risk women. According to their statement, "The NPA believes that planned home birth should be attended by a qualified practitioner within a system that provides a smooth and rapid transition to hospital if necessary." And in a recent joint statement, the Royal College of Obstetricians and Gynecologists and the Royal College of Midwives, both in the UK, said, "There is no reason why home birth should not be offered to women at low risk of complications and it may confer considerable benefits for them and their families. There is ample evidence showing that laboring at home increases a woman's likelihood of a birth that is both satisfying and safe, with implications for her health and that of her baby."

One of our advising obstetricians, Dr. Stuart Fischbein, co-author of *Fearless Pregnancy: Wisdom and Reassurance from a Doctor, a Midwife, and a Mom*, wrote to ACOG asking them to provide proof that home birth is dangerous; the doctor who responded could cite only anecdotal stories from members rather than scientific studies. That was all the proof the respondent offered to support a position that could effectively rob families of their choice in how to birth their babies. As Dr. Fischbein wrote, "Any statement saying that it is as simple as patient safety and that one-size-fits-all hospital births under the 'obstetric model' of practice should be applied to all patients is, putting it nicely, not really in line with what best serves all our patients. In many instances, hospitals are not safe, certainly not nurturing and have a far worse track record for disasters than home birth."

Despite the fact that home birth is not illegal, it sure feels like it is in some parts of this country. In many states, midwives risk prosecution if they attend a birth anywhere outside the hospital. You can have your neighbor, the FedEx delivery person, or a taxicab driver there and that's fine, but if a midwife is in the room, she could actually lose her license.

PUTTING YOUR DREAM TEAM TOGETHER

Why would you need a whole team of people around you to give birth? The one thing you do know about this whole process is that you can't be sure how everything is going to play out. Remember, Abby had planned for a natural birth at home but Matteo needed to be born in the hospital. The dash to the hospital and the emergency C-section were definitely not part of her plan. But she had surrounded herself with people who understood her wishes and who knew the hospital well. As she said, she never felt that things were happening that she wasn't informed about or that the situation was completely out of her control. Her midwife, Cara; her partner, Paulo; and Ricki were watching out for her, making sure she was protected. Her obstetrician provided the backup when it was necessary. She had a great team.

The team you assemble—even more so than the location—is key to having the kind of birth you want. You can have a beautiful natural birth in a hospital or at home depending on whom you choose to have around you and how they support your intentions. Choosing the location carefully increases your chances of getting what you want, but having a well-chosen support team ensures that, no matter what happens, you won't feel unsupported or alone.

As you consider an obstetrician and/or a midwife, you'll want to ask that person particular questions to help you understand if his or her idea of a best birth is in synch with your own. The reason you must question so carefully is that by agreeing to have your baby under this person's care, you're basically agreeing to his or her philosophy of intervention and pain management. Although this relationship evolves over time and you can always change your mind or disagree with your provider, it does help to start out with someone who can work with your goals and has the track record and statistics to prove it.

This is important because things happen pretty quickly in labor and, again, you do not want to be fighting battles with people about the care of your body when you should be focused on getting your baby out.

We know of one mom whose sister threw her body in front of the doctor to block him from cutting an episiotomy when she saw the surgical scissors were concealed behind his back. The sister knew her sibling's preferences, but the doctor didn't seem to care. Clearly this is not something you want playing out in delivery. Not only do you not want your supporters in that role (as they might not see those scissors when they're focused on you), but you also don't want a doctor who will sneak around in order to violate your personal preferences.

We'll specify those questions as we move through this section and you can choose to ask as many or as few of them that address the things you're concerned about. The caution we emphasize here is to make sure that you are really listening to the answers.

We're not your mothers telling you that you never listen. What we're talking about is a particular kind of listening, which is listening as much to yourself as it is listening to what the professionals before you have to say. These people are going to be your companions during one of the most memorable moments of your life.

You want to know that you are working with someone who is listening to you and giving you what you need in the form of attention, support, and information. Pay attention to how you feel the entire time you visit these professionals. Does the office seem warm and welcoming? Does the staff treat you with decency or are they too rushed to make this a personal exchange?

If your prospective caregiver makes you feel uncomfortable, difficult, or stupid sitting in the office, just project forward to how those same feelings will affect you on the day your child is born. The best way to find a caregiver is through women you know who have been pleased with the way they were treated during their pregnancy and birth. It is perfectly fine to decide to change a caregiver who makes you feel uncomfortable or always seems pressed for time.

As you progress along the road to your due date and start to finalize your preferences, it will become clear which of your friends and family you want to have around you, a subject we'll address later in this section. Here we want to explore the fact that there are two very different models for birth: the kind you get with most doctors and the kind you get with most midwives. Choosing one or the other—much like choosing a hospital or a birth center or a home birth—means you are unwittingly expressing a preference for a certain style of birth.

Chapter

3

Obstetricians

Finding Dr. Right

Most pregnant women sign up to have their baby with a doctor without much thought about the doctor or that office's style of practice. When they do their home pregnancy tests and see that it's positive, most women inform their gynecologists and arrange for care with that doctor or another in the practice who works in obstetrics, even though when they embark on pregnancy, they might see their doctors with different eyes and evaluate them according to different standards.

When Childbirth Connections surveyed thousands of women for their Listening to Mothers II survey, they asked them how they chose their doctor. Most said they simply picked the one covered by their insurance and 83 percent didn't visit any others to see if a different doctor might be a better fit. We're trained by insurance companies—and the experiences of our friends who have had babies—not to expect that much from obstetrical services. And there's good reason not to get too excited.

You wait forever in the waiting room for your exam, then sit forlornly freezing in your little paper gown in the glaring examination room when (surprise!) the doctor who comes to examine you is one you've never seen before. He has to look at your chart to figure out your name. You can be excused for feeling like you're on a conveyor belt toward birth. Laid out on that crackly paper with a complete stranger poking around your most intimate parts, it's hard not to feel that this significant moment in your life is pretty insignificant.

Mostly it's not the doctor's fault. Doctors survive in a high-pressure system where it's tough for them to make a living. Most obstetricians have to work half the year just to pay their malpractice premiums. They actively manage your labor with a style of defensive medicine, meaning care that their insurance company can defend in a lawsuit.

From the perspective of a woman who is very concerned about risks, this can be reassuring. The deepening pile of results from the tests they order seems to predict a medically correct outcome for her and her baby. But it's a style of care that puts the test results ahead of the personal touch and what the woman's body might be telling her. The active style of pregnancy management requires more testing, which results in more inductions, more C-sections, no VBACs, and a phobia about allowing women who are having large babies to birth naturally. The factors combine to make doctors see your pregnancy as a constant state of crisis and your body as an unpredictable mechanism that is just about to malfunction.

The financial and legal pressures on obstetricians are enormous. Every minute they spend answering your questions is a minute they aren't spending with money-making patients in the other rooms. This is probably why many doctors trained in obstetrics and gynecology only practice obstetrics for a few years and move in mid-career to the better hours and more manageable risks of plain gynecology. For many it's a terrible disappointment. They started in this specialty because they loved helping women have their babies. The way obstetricians are trained and the legal environment they practice in gets them further and further away from their original expectation of being a doctor.

Megan Callahan was just out of medical school at the University of Virginia and rotating through the different disciplines trying to choose a specialty. The first stop was obstetrics and, after the first delivery she witnessed, she couldn't think of doing anything else. "It's so joyful and the connection with the patient is so strong," said Dr. Callahan, who is now in her first year of practice in Seattle. "Every delivery is different. You can't help, no matter what time it is, no matter what is going on, feeling that joy."

Then the training to become an obstetrician began.

The first stop in her four-year residency was a year spent on normal birth. Unfortunately Megan didn't see too many normal births. The population she served at her teaching hospital was mainly poor people. Many women she saw were coming in for their first prenatal appointments far into their pregnancies and carried with them a host of health problems. This meant that Dr. Callahan's study of normal pregnancy focused on patients who presented complications like diabetes, morbid obesity, and high blood pressure. After that, Dr. Callahan and her fellow residents completed three years of rigorous study of everything that can go wrong in pregnancy and labor. Abby's obstetrician Dr. Jacques Moritz, who trained at Columbia University thirty years ago and now teaches there, says he remembers only seeing one or two "normal" births during his residency.

"We were taking care of people who did not have a lot of resources," Dr. Callahan said. "Birth is not always a joyful experience for people who do not have the extra money to feed this child."

As Dr. Callahan says, we want our doctors to know all there is to know about abnormal pregnancy. That's what we pay them for. But when you consider the way that doctors are trained to think about pregnancy, you can see why many see it as a crisis that requires management and monitoring. The doctor must be active and vigilant for any indication that your birth is starting to move into dangerous territory. At any moment something could go wrong. To monitor the crisis, the doctor needs the technology, technicians, and interventions that are only available at the hospital. With this basic philosophy as the starting point, doctors tend to oppose anyone who considers giving birth outside the hospital.

Firing Your Caregiver, Even If You're Thirty Weeks Along

It's horrifying to say this, but even when women are pregnant many of us are still people pleasers. Many women, in telling the story of when their birth took a wrong turn, explain how they didn't want to bother the nurse or how they felt bad waking the doctor. One woman told us that she agreed to stop pushing because the staff was tired and there was about to be a shift change. She didn't want them being cranky at the birth. So, given that, how can you get the guts to fire your caregiver?

Dr. Staci Emerson, a Los Angeles psychologist, did and it made all the difference in the birth of her second son.

At thirty weeks, Staci's doctor told her that he could not promise her a private room, that is, one that would allow her husband to attend, for the birth unless she scheduled a daytime induction. This was so different from what she wanted that she decided to find out about midwives, an option she'd never considered before.

At the first visit to her hospital birth center, she was so inspired by the idea of women-centered care that she signed a contract on the spot and paid up front in full. Shortly after that, she discovered that she and her midwife did not get along.

She had expected a warm and informal atmosphere. Instead her midwife wore a white coat just like a doctor. Staci had a lot of questions, of course, transferring at such a late stage in her pregnancy. But when she asked them, her midwife made her feel like a dumb and pesky little girl. For example, when she asked for the name of the doctor who would be backing up the midwife in the hospital if she had to transfer out of the birth center, the midwife said sternly that she wouldn't give Staci that information. Those were her relationships, not Staci's.

Staci left the birth center in tears. At the third meeting, when Staci started crying again, the midwife told her, "This is the way I do things. If you want a healthy baby and you want this baby to survive, you are going to have to do what I tell you to do."

(continued)

When Staci got home, she asked her husband to come with her to the next prenatal visit so that she could get his support in firing the midwife. He was very skeptical, thinking that there was something wrong with Staci, not the midwife, because she was demanding to make another change so late in the pregnancy. As they walked out of the birth center after the visit, her husband said he supported her completely in her choice.

Still Staci worried that she was making a stressful situation even worse. She talked about her anxiety and indecision with her doula and many of the pregnant women she knew. "I have a best friend who will always tell me the truth. So, when she validated and supported my experience, I felt so much better about my choice," Staci said.

Staci found another midwife who was more suited to her temperament. "I called her on the phone and I fell in love with her," she said. "What I was asking for was so simple. I wanted someone to root for me. She came to my house the next day and we spent three hours together." The midwife, Susan Gill, supported Staci in a home birth. She gave birth to her son after a three-hour labor in a birthing tub set up in her bedroom.

"He was born twelve hours before my oldest's birthday," Staci noted. "Had I been in the hospital I would have had to tell him that I was sorry we couldn't have his birthday party. Instead my midwife and my husband and my sons and I were all bouncing around in the jumpy house we had set up for the party the next day. I had sixty people in my house and they were saying, 'You just had a baby?'"

The irony of the fact that she is a psychologist who specializes in working with women who have body image issues was not lost on Staci. "My intuition was telling me the other people were wrong and I was frightened to go with that," Staci said. "Everything Susan taught me was to listen to my body, touch my body, and hear what it was saying to me."

If your pregnancy is complicated or risky or the baby is genuinely in distress, the doctors can use their expertise to ensure a safe delivery for your baby. They deliver babies who would not have had a chance even forty years ago. Yet there is a downside to having so much expertise.

The old saying is, when you have a hammer in your hand, everything looks like a nail. If you apply that aphorism to doctors, when they have all these incredibly cool medical tools, they're looking for a way to use them.

Former director of the World Health Organization maternal and child health division Dr. Marsden Wagner compares having an obstetrician oversee a normal childbirth to hiring a child psychiatrist as a babysitter. You'll come home from an evening out to find that the shrink has diagnosed your spirited child as having an oppositional personality disorder that requires special drugs and therapy. This would be the psychiatric model of babysitting, similar to the medical model of childbirth.

At first Dr. Callahan, who is now in her first year of practice, was surprised by the patients she treated in another part of Seattle. These moms were so different from those she served in her residency. They came to the prenatal visits having read books, researched pregnancy on the Internet, and embarked on yoga and special diets that promised to keep them and their babies in the best of health.

As a reflective young person still trying to get a handle on what kind of doctor she will be, Dr. Callahan often shows the heart rate monitor strips from births she's attended to the more experienced doctors in the practice and compares their reading of them to her own thoughts. "What I want to give the parents is a perfectly healthy and totally intact child who can live to the best of his or her potential," she said. "That's what I struggle with. When is the baby not doing well? When is the baby going to benefit from a C-section? When does an intervention result in a better outcome for mom and baby?"

Even with all her talent, skill, and empathy, she too has to be mindful of the legal climate. She and the doctors in her practice do VBACs, but they do not do breech deliveries after a 2000 article in the *New England Journal of Medicine* showed an increased risk to breech babies from a vaginal delivery. "The problem with practicing in the U.S. is once you have an article that is well done in a well-respected journal and you have a bad outcome in a birth, you do not stand a chance in trial," she said.

Using a Family Physician for Your Birth

You may not know that you can actually use a family physician for your birth. Some women have great experiences with this.

The cornerstone of family medicine is the belief that all people should have a personal patient–physician relationship focused on integrated care. In maternity care, this means that your personal physician cares for you and your family through the transitions of pregnancy, birth, and parenting. Family physician Wendy Brooks Barr, MD, MPH, MSCE, explains, "Most family physicians who provide maternity care provide prenatal care to low- or moderate-risk patients and attend vaginal deliveries, similar to midwives. They work with either obstetricians or family physicians with additional operative and high-risk obstetrical training who assist them if a complication arises that requires a C-section or other surgical procedure. Some family physicians receive additional training in high-risk obstetrics and cesarean sections and can care for high-risk patients. There are also family physicians who provide office-based prenatal care only and then work with a group of midwives or obstetricians who attend the delivery. All of these family physicians then care for the newborn in addition to the woman after delivery and continue to provide primary care for all members of the family. Many women find it easier to develop a high level of trust and comfort with their pediatric provider if that same provider was involved in their maternity care."

According to the Listening to Mothers II survey, family physicians attend approximately 8 percent of births in the United States. The number is typically lower in major urban areas and much higher in rural areas where family physicians attend a large percentage of births and are an important resource for women to continue to have access to local maternity care. Multiple studies have shown that family physicians provide high-quality maternity care for low-risk patients. As compared to obstetrician-specialists, family physicians often have lower practice-based rates of episiotomy, vacuum/forceps delivery, and cesarean delivery.

If you adore your family physician, consider making him or her your primary caregiver for your birth. Or if you've heard great things about a local family physician, think about including this doctor in your interview process as you seek out your primary caregiver.

Speaking of that same study, New York obstetrician Dr. Eden Fromberg said the reaction to it demonstrates how cynical the profession has become about letting women make their own choices and doctors use all their skills. She calls it the "lost art of obstetrics," meaning many doctors are no longer delivering twins or breeches or using forceps even if they are the best tool for turning the baby in the birth canal because of the legal risk, not the situation of the baby or the mother.

What doctors hold out as a trade-off from making all the choices is the false guarantee of absolute safety for you and your baby as delivered via machines. "We're not giving people options and not trusting that people can make decisions," Dr. Fromberg said. "What if you say to a woman that there is a one in eight chance of some trouble in a vaginal breech delivery? One woman might focus on the fact that that risk sounds pretty high to her and choose a C-section. Another might say that seven out of eight successes are pretty good odds."

Many doctors simply tell women that they are having a C-section, rather than consulting with them first.

"The business of medicine is awfully coercive," said Dr. Stuart Fischbein, a Los Angeles obstetrician. "Hospital risk managers and insurance companies are making the decisions that affect the lives of patients who they never have to look in the eye. We are training doctors to be sheep, not shepherds. One successful lawsuit can devastate the hospital's bottom line for years, so there is pressure to protect the hospital from liability, despite what the hospital's television commercials tell you."

Dr. Fischbein, who trained twenty-five years ago at a Los Angeles County hospital that did sixty-five births a day, had significant contact with patients but now sees how distant the practice of obstetrics has become for newly trained doctors. Dr. Moritz remembers that when he was a resident, he was required to pop in every ten minutes to take a look at laboring women. Now the doctors at the hospital manage their patients "more centrally" and spend a significant amount of time learning the technology. At the hospital where he practices, a resident sits in front of two plasma screens monitoring the readings from the various electronic devices affixed to the mothers and plotting their progress on graphs "like an air traffic controller at JFK."

Questions for Your Doctor

- If you are unavailable when I'm in labor, what is your plan for a backup? Can I meet that doctor or doctors before my due date?
- At what point in labor will you arrive?
- Do you allow a doula, midwife, and/or friends and family to be present while I am in labor?
- What kind of prenatal testing do you normally recommend?
- Do you encourage movement and positioning during labor?
- Which hospitals do you have privileges at? Can I choose whatever hospital I like?
- How much fetal monitoring do you do during labor?
- What is your C-section rate? Under what circumstances do you recommend a C-section?
- How often do you cut episiotomies? How often do you opt for a natural vaginal tear?
- How many of your clients deliver their babies without medication?
- How often do you use forceps or vacuum extraction?
- How many of your clients are induced? How long past the due date do you allow them to go before scheduling an induction?
- Right after my baby is born, what is the normal routine? Will I be able to hold my baby immediately?

This is the high-tech, low-touch method of childbearing. So you can understand why, when you pull out a long list of questions designed to establish the doctor's style of care, many times he or she has one eye on you and one eye on the clock. The pressure of that can make doctors brusque. They might start to see you as a troublemaker because maintaining malpractice insurance and following the protocols of the hospital restrict the kind of care they can give you.

That said, you have a right to find out what kind of practice your doctor prefers. It's best not to ask these questions in the middle of your examination. Sit down with your doctor face-to-face so you can concentrate on the answers and body language. Make sure you get the specifics.

If your doctor says her C-section rate is "in line with the national average," you know from reading this book that the national average is close to a third of all births. What you really want to know is under which conditions she insists a woman have a C-section and, if she is in a group practice, what the C-section average is for the group. If you have become a patient at a large group practice of four or more doctors, there is a very good chance that the doctor who delivers your baby will not be the one you have grown to think of as your doctor. Do not assume that because you've chosen a woman doctor she will be less likely to intervene in your birth, if that's what you're after. Men and women go through the same training in medical school, and the way they become doctors is a transformative experience. You've got to ask everybody you meet the right questions in preparation for your best birth.

Birth Goddess: Laila Ali

Athlete Laila Ali's birth of her first child wasn't as she planned it. "Things didn't go exactly how I would have liked them to have gone," she said, "but I still believe they went as they were supposed to." Although Laila didn't have the natural birth she initially envisioned, she had a vaginal birth, and she had a birth team that balanced her wishes and the baby's well-being. Laila believes that she made smart choices as each option was presented to her along the way.

Laila had planned for a natural birth at home. "My thing is, I always want to be in control," Laila said. "I didn't want anyone doing anything to me or my child that wasn't necessary, for reasons that have to do with wanting to get out of the hospital early, wanting to go home, wanting you to have a fast labor, or wanting to make money. Those were the things I didn't want to have anything to do with. Those were the things that I learned went on in

(continued)

the medical industry, so that's why I was like, 'I want to do this naturally and I want to do it at home.' "

When Laila was five months along, a sonogram revealed that the baby might be experiencing a growth restriction (they later found that the umbilical cord was too short and the placenta was calcified). The midwives she'd been working with were no longer comfortable with Laila's birthing the baby at home. It was then that Laila understood she'd need to have a hospital birth. Ten days before her due date, although he couldn't yet pinpoint exactly what the problem was, her doctor told her that the conditions for the baby were better on the outside than they were on the inside. He gave her the options of being induced that day or waiting a few more days. "I prayed and listened to everyone's advice, went with what was in my heart, and I said, 'Let's go ahead and do this now,' " she said. She was nervous about getting Pitocin because she knew that meant the contractions would be much harder, but she felt she should do whatever she needed to do.

After the Pitocin was administered, Laila labored for fourteen hours, and was still only dilated a few centimeters. "My doctor said it could take another six to seven hours. I didn't know if I was going to be able to handle it," she said. Laila hadn't eaten or had anything to drink for hours, and she was in a lot of pain. She felt like she was going to faint, and she was exhausted. "I knew then that I should get an epidural. I kept asking everyone in the room, 'Are you going to be disappointed in me if I do that?' Everyone said, 'No, go ahead, get it,' " she said.

"Once I got the epidural, I thought 'Man, this is easy!' When it came time to push, I was ready. I remembered what my doctor had said about how to push, and I was like, 'I'm going to do this the way they told me to do it, and focus on that.' I felt pressure, even though I didn't feel pain. I was still connected enough. It took twenty-three minutes and six contractions, and the baby was out," Laila said.

Because Laila had the epidural, she was able to avoid having a C-section. Her husband, Curtis, actually caught the baby. "When CJ came out, his eyes were open, so I was like, 'Man, he probably couldn't see me, but I felt like I was the first person he laid eyes on when he entered the world.' That was really special for me. When you have an experience like that, your emotions just take over your body. Inside, I was trembling. I was going a hundred miles an hour," Curtis said.

Laila added, "At that moment, nothing mattered anymore. Everything was in the past. You just have to go with the flow. In the end, all that matters is that you have a healthy baby. I feel really blessed to have the baby here, and everything about him is perfect now. I have my perfect baby."

Chapter
4

Midwives
Not Just for Hippies Anymore

Midwives are burdened by an unfortunate reputation as folk medicine kooks who are not medically trained. The reality is very far from that. Both of us worked with midwives to birth our children. Getting to know midwives and seeing how competent and dedicated they are was one of the most meaningful discoveries we made on our paths to motherhood.

Generally midwives approach the care of pregnant women as a collaboration between two equals, with the midwife pledged to fully informing you and advising you in the decisions you are going to make about your prenatal care and plans for the birth. They practice what some have described as the low-tech, high-touch method of care. Midwives see pregnancy as a natural process that, for most women, needs no intervention. The term midwife is an old one that means "with woman," which seems apt. A good midwife is centered on you and with you all the way through your pregnancy, something that is missing from most modern obstetrical care.

If you've engaged the services of a home birth midwife, she might come to your home for prenatal visits. (If you're working with a doctor who has a midwife on staff, you'll see her for your prenatal care at the doctor's office. The rule of thumb is that a prenatal visit with a home birth midwife lasts from forty-five to sixty minutes; with a hospital-based midwife the visit is from fifteen to twenty minutes; and with a doctor it is from five to six minutes.)

As we know, midwives can also work in independent hospital-based practices, clinics, and birth centers. Many nurse-midwives have hospital privileges, which means they can deliver babies in a particular hospital. A nurse-midwife with hospital privileges has a strong relationship with the hospital. By granting her privileges, the staff and the physicians are acknowledging that they know her work style and respect her, which can ease her clients' navigation through the hospital system.

Midwives with independent practices are usually affiliated with a large hospital. In Ricki's first pregnancy, she was the patient of a midwifery service affiliated with St. Luke's–Roosevelt Hospital in New York City. When she came to the office for her visits, she would see any of the midwives on staff. The midwives in a group practice do this so that if you go into labor when a different one of them is on call, you will feel comfortable and familiar with all the midwives in the practice. For Ricki's second pregnancy she chose a midwife who attended the birth of her baby at home.

When it comes to normal, vaginal births, midwives are the experts, even though obstetricians have similar skills for normal births. Many obstetricians would agree that midwives are essentially more skilled at normal deliveries because that is the focus of their training. If you are a patient in a private midwifery practice that delivers babies in a hospital or hospital birth center, you will go to their professional offices, have the same exact schedule of prenatal appointments as you would with an obstetrician, have the same tests ordered (sonograms, amnio, etc.), and have all of this covered by insurance if the midwives take your plan. They will also support you if you choose not to have an ultrasound or genetic testing.

The difference is that midwives take on fewer patients so they can spend more time with them at each appointment. Prenatal appointments with midwives, which can start as early as eight weeks into pregnancy, are generally longer, more comprehensive, and more personal. They tend to focus on more holistic care, caring for the whole woman, which in addition to your physical health means asking you about your diet and your relationships, the stresses you're feeling, and what is going on at work and with your kids. The process is personal and intuitive as well as medical, tailored to the woman's individual needs.

Besides this personal touch, they have other ways to make you feel less like a patient. You may find oven mitts over the metal stirrups on the exam table! Sometimes you will weigh yourself in the bathroom when you give your urine sample and then write it down on your own chart instead of having a nurse weigh you like a child. (This is always the *worst* moment of every prenatal appointment!) They may have couches and beanbags in their office so you aren't sitting on the exam chair when you and the midwife talk.

Midwives: Two Choices

There are two kinds of professionally trained midwives: the certified nurse-midwife and the certified professional midwife.

Certified nurse-midwife. A CNM has qualified as a registered nurse and completed an additional two years of graduate work focusing specifically on pregnancy and birth. Most of these midwives practice in hospitals or birth centers, although some do home births if having a nurse-midwife present at a home birth is legal in that state. If they work on their own, either in a midwifery practice or by running a birth center, they do so in collaboration with or under the supervision of a doctor.

Certified professional midwife. This kind of midwife has studied pregnancy and birth formally through a program that does not require a nurse certificate. In order to get her credential, she needs to verify that she has completed the required clinical training, which includes attending births and doing prenatal care. Currently, most of these midwives attend births at home.

The other difference is that when you show up at the hospital in labor, the midwife will meet you there and help you in labor, unlike the physician, who is called in at the last minute. Once in the hospital, the midwives can do *anything* a physician can do except C-sections, vacuum or forceps-assisted deliveries, and repairing third- or fourth-degree tears (meaning a tear from vagina to anus). Midwives can arrange for an epidural, administer pain medications, induce labor, give an episiotomy if necessary, or repair a natural vaginal tear. (Most women don't realize that they can have an epidural and still work with a midwife.) Many circumcise baby boys if the parents choose. They can also call for a C-section and often work with a collaborating doctor, whom you can meet before the birth so you are acquainted if you develop complications during labor. Your midwife can be by your side if you have a C-section.

During labor, midwives generally tend to minimize the use of technology. Their favored technique for helping labor progress is to let the woman's body find its own rhythm. They and the doulas they work with have witnessed enough childbirths that they can detect when things are getting moving. Part of their monitoring is to advise moms to shift into positions and take actions that help ease the pain. They stand quietly on the alert for signs of distress and will act swiftly if medical intervention is needed. Their training includes identifying when a woman needs a doctor's help either in pregnancy or labor. If you work with a midwife at a home birth or a birth center, she will be prepared to oversee the birth and transfer you to the hospital for necessary interventions.

Ivy League Midwives

Carolyn Havens Niemann came from a family of academics. She followed her father's, grandfather's, and great-grandfather's footsteps and enrolled at Princeton University after finishing high school. While at Princeton, she took a course on women's history where she first learned about the shift from home birth to hospital birth. "The professor talked about birth changing from a central focus of the 'women's sphere' to something essentially controlled

(continued)

by men," Carolyn said. "I became interested in midwifery from a historical and feminist perspective." That same semester, her favorite professor at Princeton gave birth to her third child in an out-of-hospital birth center with midwives. "I had no idea until that point that modern midwives existed. It had never crossed my mind to question our current system of maternity care until this woman, who was one of the first female faculty members with tenure at Princeton, made a choice to give birth in this way."

Leslie Turner chose to become a midwife after graduating from Yale University with a bachelor's degree in psychology. "I was drawn to the study of medicine, yet I was very interested in the field of psychology. Becoming a midwife involved the marriage of both disciplines." Like Carolyn, Leslie had very little exposure to the profession. "I was surprised to discover that the vast majority of midwives work in hospitals, side by side with obstetricians, anesthesiologists, and neonatologists. Modern midwifery embraces technology, while still preserving the profession's focus on partnering with the patient."

After graduation Carolyn worked as a minimally paid birth assistant in the same birth center where her professor had given birth. "I still believe that a huge amount of what I know today I learned during that first year. I was privileged to attend ten deliveries during that first year, the first of which was a ten-and-a-half-pound baby born in a standing squat in a doorway over an intact perineum (meaning, there was no cut or tear in the area of tissue and muscle between the anus and vagina). I knew that this was not how most women in America were delivering their babies."

Soon after that, Carolyn witnessed her first hospital birth. "The woman was twenty-six and giving birth to her sixth child. She was deep in the throes of labor in a room shared with three other women. The obstetrical resident came in to put a fetal scalp electrode on the baby's head to monitor the fetal heart rate. She resisted, and he said to her, 'Shut your mouth and open your legs.' I was horrified. This, of course, was why she was twenty-six and having her sixth child. All her life she had probably been told to shut her mouth and open her legs."

Because Leslie had decided to become a midwife after graduating from

Yale, she had to go back to school to obtain the prerequisite science courses she had not previously taken and then attended Columbia University to obtain her master's degree with a dual specialty as a midwife and women's health nurse-practitioner. In addition to long hours in the classroom, there were countless days and nights in the hospital gaining clinical experience, and then many more hours spent studying for the board certification exam. Going back to school involved a huge commitment of time, energy, and money.

Carolyn attended midwifery school at the University of California, San Francisco, and also found it extremely challenging. "The three-year program of midwifery study was incredibly rigorous; I was surprised to find that I had to work much harder during the initial year, which was a condensed year of nursing school, than I ever had at Princeton." After graduation Carolyn was offered a position as a midwife in a community clinic in Harlem. "The commitment was for two years, but I stayed for four and learned more than I thought I possibly could about medicine, midwifery, and myself." In fact, Carolyn ended up having her very own ten-and-a-half-pound home birth over an intact perineum!

Now practicing in New York City, Leslie finds great reward in working with women of all ages: "While most people think about a midwife in the role of attending births, in actuality it is so much more. Midwives are trained to work with women throughout the lifespan, far beyond their reproductive years. While I love providing family planning and prenatal care and attending births, my work with postmenopausal women is so enriching. In my current position I work with women of all ages, from thirteen to ninety, as well as all races and backgrounds. Being a midwife is about so much more than assisting a woman through the process of birth. It is about assisting a woman through the process of life; providing her with information and a safe space to make choices that support her physical, emotional, and social health."

For Carolyn, one of the most interesting things has been to watch her Princeton classmates' reactions to her career choice over the years: "At my

(continued)

fifth reunion at Princeton, my classmates looked at me quizzically when I told them I had just graduated from midwifery school. Most of them had headed directly from Princeton to law school, business school, or medical school. Fast-forward to the tenth reunion, and I was greeted with far less skepticism. By the fifteenth reunion, classmates were actually flocking to me, eager to relay their birth stories. These were divided into two categories: those who had chosen to deliver with a doctor, had had a bad experience, and promised me that the next time they were going straight to their local midwife, and those who had done their homework ahead of time and had delivered with midwives."

Leslie has no regrets about not pursuing a medical career. "Birth is truly the most amazing experience a human being can ever witness. This is where the magic of midwifery unfolds, the sacred bond between midwife and mother is created. A woman is at her most vulnerable, yet also her most courageous, during the process of birth. To witness the beginning of a life, to guide that life safely into this world is an awe-inspiring responsibility and blessing."

Carolyn agrees. "I have great respect for my peers who have chosen medical school; thank goodness we have committed, well-educated physicians when we need them. But as the guardians of normal birth, we midwives need just as much to attract bright and eager young people to our profession to carry on a tradition as old as birth itself."

Midwives aren't as concerned that labor follow a certain timeline, but they are aware of when it may be going on too long for the safety of the baby and the mother's level of energy and tolerance for pain. They understand that sometimes an intervention like an epidural or Pitocin can actually help a woman avoid a C-section in a hospital setting by facilitating her labor. Ultimately a midwife wants to empower you to push your own baby out safely and she will be there to "catch" it. Midwives don't like to use the word "deliver" as this takes away from the mother's active participation in the birth.

Midwifery Underground

Nurse-midwives are legal in every state but certified professional midwives are licensed/regulated in only twenty-six states. Some states actively prosecute midwives or have laws on the books that make practicing midwifery illegal as the unauthorized practice of medicine or nursing, which would be considered either a felony or misdemeanor under that state's law. This means that having your baby at home is not illegal in any state, but if you live in a state where certified professional midwives (CPMs) cannot legally practice and a CPM attends the birth, she might be prosecuted. As with other professions such as doctors, lawyers, and teachers, if a CPM is licensed in one state, that license is not valid in a different state.

The American Medical Association has begun a new campaign to get state boards of medicine to crack down on all unlicensed practitioners. So unless a state licenses midwives, their legal status remains unsafe.

The Big Push for Midwives is a national campaign that is working to win laws that allow CPMs to be licensed and that make sure their services are regulated in all fifty states. Requiring CPMs to pass a national license exam, continue their education on an ongoing basis, and be subject to peer review and state regulation would enhance consumer confidence in the profession. The Big Push recently won a victory in Missouri where the state supreme court upheld a law legalizing CPMs, thereby overturning a challenge by a state physicians' group. The plight of CPMs in the United States is unfortunate, because many women have had excellent results using a CPM at their home birth. Check out your state's guidelines at the Big Push for Midwives site listed in the Resources section at the back of this book if you're interested in hiring a CPM.

If you have a high-risk pregnancy, the doctor's vigilance and careful management of all the factors can save the lives of you and your baby. If you are convinced that the only safe place to have a baby is in the hospital, a freestanding birth center or a home birth would not be the right choice for you. The last thing you need when you're going into labor is to be stiff with doubts about whether you made a good choice.

Seems like a wonderful division of labor, doesn't it? The midwives handle the pregnancies that do not require the attention of specialists and surgeons, leaving those doctors free to do what they do best. This is the way pregnancy is managed all across Europe and Japan, where midwives attend 70 percent of the normal deliveries while they attend less than 11 percent in this country. Mary Breckinridge's story helps explain why the American system is so unbalanced. You'd think that doctors and midwives would be on the same team, united in wanting to help women have the best births possible. In fact, historically, they are engaged in a turf war over what constitutes good maternity care, and it is a struggle that has been going on for more than a century.

Birth Goddess: Mary Breckinridge

Mary Breckinridge almost single-handedly saved midwifery when the medical profession was trying to stamp it out in the 1920s. She was a rich woman, the granddaughter of a former Kentucky governor, and had been trained as a nurse. She found herself alone at midlife after both of her children died young and she and her husband divorced.

Mary decided to do what she could for the mothers of Appalachia. She set off on her horse through the mountains, crisscrossing the fields and the streams, and saw girls who were fourteen years old still working the land when they were in their ninth month of pregnancy. She also met the granny midwives who had been so demonized by the obstetricians. She decided that professional midwifery was the answer to this health care crisis, but she needed to get more training to prove this.

Mary went to the United Kingdom for midwifery training, which was illegal in the United States. When she returned to Kentucky in 1925, she brought with her some of the graduates from midwifery school, who were intrigued by this wild adventure. Mary believed that if she was going to make a dent in the public health crisis there, she had to start treating babies and follow them into adulthood. Her Frontier Nursing Service established health outposts in remote areas of Appalachia and the midwives set to work. In the backcountry, these scandalous women wore trousers (!) and sheepskin coats and carried snakebite serum with them.

Mary knew that if she was going to prove the value of this work, she had to keep verifiable records, which she had tabulated by the Metropolitan Life Insurance Company. In its first report on the FNS, the company praised Mary's methods, saying that if her techniques were used nationwide, they would save "10,000 mothers' lives per year in the United States, there would be 30,000 less still births and 30,000 more children alive at the end of the first month of life." The company recommended widespread training of midwives. In 1939, a time when midwifery was all but nonexistent in the United States, Mary founded the Frontier Graduate School of Midwifery.

In the FNS's first thirty years, the nurse-midwives attended more than ten thousand births. All maternal and infant outcome statistics were better than for the country as a whole. In the poorest part of the country, the FNS's maternal mortality rate was nine per ten thousand births compared with thirty-four per ten thousand for the United States as a whole.

The story of Mary and her Frontier Nursing Service spread to urban capitals, inspiring nursing schools to start up an effort to get nurse-midwives certified. The first nurse-midwifery program was established in New York City in 1931 and Columbia-Presbyterian Hospital founded a program in 1955, the first to certify nurses in obstetrics. Midwives gradually started to reclaim respectability, and in 1971 the American College of Obstetricians and Gynecologists agreed that midwives were competent to attend uncomplicated births. Within a few years, nurse-midwives were legal in every state. Although Mary died in 1965, Frontier Nursing Service exists to this day, still serving the mothers of Appalachia in a hospital named after its founder.

Today we are in the midst of a resurgence of interest in natural childbirth and midwifery, particularly as a backlash to an overmedicalized maternity system.

A century ago there was a huge class divide in the way babies were born. Middle- and upper-class women were attended by family physicians and poor women had midwives, some of whom had studied in professional midwifery school and others who had practical experience.

As families were moving from the country into the cities with their big hospitals, people began to embrace birth governed by technology. Suffragettes who were campaigning for women's rights thought that getting pain relief for childbirth was a feminist issue and narcotics were only available in the hospital. It's hard to escape the other feminist issue in this dispute—the doctors who oversaw the technological hospital birth were nearly all male and midwifery was an exclusively female world run by strong and feisty women who felt no need to have male doctors around at childbirth.

In 1910 the Carnegie Foundation issued a report critical of all medical training in the United States and singling out obstetrics for the most criticism. Obstetricians of that era did not even have to graduate from high school to be admitted into an obstetrics program and the course work didn't include laboratory or clinical training. The report also found a great need for prenatal care, which was not common then.

Ironically, obstetricians used the report to promote the idea that midwives made birth unsafe. They created a campaign to discredit midwives and drive birth into the hospital. Magazines depicted midwives as poor and uneducated, implying that the care they provided was inferior and unsafe.

In addition to this smear campaign against midwives, there were also legal prosecutions. Dr. Marsden Wagner, former head of the World Health Organization maternal and fetal health division, cites the case of midwife Hanna Porn from Gardner, Massachusetts, who in 1905 was sentenced to prison for practicing medicine without a license, although she had completed a six-month program at the Chicago Midwife Institute. There were no licenses for midwives in Massachusetts at that time. Despite her lack of nursing credentials, the births Hanna Porn attended had lower stillbirth and neonatal mortality rates than those of the doctors. The state used Hanna Porn's case, among others, as a justification for criminalizing midwifery and other states followed Massachusetts's lead. Until the 1950s and the rise of certified nurse-midwives, midwifery was banned in nearly all fifty states.

This campaign forced midwifery underground until it battled back in the middle of the last century. Smarting from the blow of being marginalized by doctors, midwives decided they needed to have professional certificates that legitimized their work. Professional midwife programs allowed nurses to add another two years onto their education and become certified nurse-midwives. By the 1980s the Carnegie Foundation report officially advocated midwifery.

Myths about Midwives

They are untrained and unprofessional. Certified nurse-midwives are nurses who must go to two years of additional training and certification to practice. Yale and Columbia Universities both have midwifery schools. Certified professional midwives have didactic and clinical education and training in birth and birth education but do not get the nursing degree.

They are only for new-agers and hippies. Midwives practice all over the United States, including in major cities like New York where clients include educated, professional women who are sold on the great benefits midwives have to offer. As Chicago midwife Amy Willen said, "I do a lot of ladies in the suburbs who drive minivans and go to soccer practice. We have such a wide variety that it boggles my mind: teachers, lawyers, dentists, nurses."

They deliver babies only at home. Ninety-eight percent of nurse-midwives work delivering babies in hospitals.

They use unconventional practices. Midwives are medically trained and conversant in the latest technology, but many are also open to nonmedical and natural solutions to childbirth problems. Midwives in out-of-hospital settings often use alternative therapies including homeopathic remedies, herbs, and acupuncture, which are increasingly being included in research studies to prove their effectiveness. Flexibility is important to their woman-centered practice.

(continued)

They are interested in promoting only fully natural childbirth. Midwives accommodate different childbirth plans, including advising women who are exhausted that labor could progress more smoothly with an epidural. If you want a natural childbirth, you are more likely to get one if your caregiver is a midwife, but they also attend hospital births with epidurals and other interventions.

Births supervised by them are more dangerous than those supervised by doctors. When normal births with doctors and midwives are compared, the midwives' patients have fewer C-sections and interventions. They specialize in normal childbirth, which affects these numbers because doctors handle a higher percentage of difficult and risky pregnancies.

They don't work with doctors. Most midwives work with collaborating doctors.

Although the number of midwives and respect for them has grown dramatically in the last thirty years, the profession has never really recovered from the smear campaign that discredited it. Midwives are still the experts on normal birth, yet they are often regulated to second-class citizenship in the world of birth.

State laws make them subordinate to doctors and all states require nurse-midwives to work under doctor supervision. Some states require that doctors approve their decision making, while others prefer a collaborative arrangement in which the midwife consults the doctor when necessary. Most midwives work with collaborating doctors. Nurse-midwives can write prescriptions, for example, but insurance companies will not allow them to order tests on their own. In order to give their clients ultrasounds or order blood work, a doctor's name has to be on the top of the order slip.

A growing number of physicians work in collaboration with midwives either by hiring them in their obstetrical practices or by working alongside them in hospital maternity wards that offer a midwifery service.

Whether or not an insurance company will reimburse you for any money you spend out of pocket for a midwife depends very much on the insurance company and on its idea of how your interaction with the midwife should be governed. For example, Judi Tinkelenberg, a CNM in California, will not accept Blue Cross insurance because it requires that a doctor be present in the room when she delivers the baby, something that is not necessary at her birth center.

More and more insurance companies, however, are covering the services of midwives, and in some states they also cover the services of CPMs in home births. Ask ahead of time so that you know what your maternity deductible will be and approximately how much to expect in reimbursement. CPMs charge between $3,000 and $6,500 for a home birth, depending on the prevailing rates in the area. Nurse-midwives typically charge a similar fee, and again, it may be covered or partially covered by your insurance carrier. Be sure to ask about rates and coverage when you interview midwives.

We feel that midwives often don't get the credit they deserve, and we urge you to keep an open mind about using midwifery services for your pregnancy. Our birth experiences would not have been what they were without our relationships with our midwives.

Questions for Your Midwife

Pregnant women often go midwife shopping! This involves calling some potential midwives that you have heard about through word-of-mouth, the Internet, or even the yellow pages. If you are still interested after a few initial questions on the phone, you can set up an introductory interview where you will meet and talk some more. Often this initial interview is free and lasts about an hour. Make sure you ask all of your questions, especially if you are planning a birth in an out-of-hospital setting. Your initial interaction with a

(continued)

midwife will oftentimes let you know if you feel comfortable with her style of care.

Here are some questions to ask:

- When do you cut an episiotomy? If the answer is that she only does that when necessary, it's important to get her idea of when it is necessary and her estimation of what percentage of women she's attended in the last year have had episiotomies.
- Are you certified? (Certified nurse-midwives and certified professional midwives should be able to produce proof of that.)
- If you are unavailable when I'm in labor, what is your plan for a backup? Can I meet that person or persons before my due date?
- Do you work with a doctor? Can I meet that doctor?
- What is your fee, and what kind of insurance do you accept?
- At what point in labor will you be with me?
- Do you allow a doula and/or friends and family to be present while a woman is in labor?
- What kind of prenatal testing do you normally recommend?
- Do you encourage movement and positioning during labor?
- If this is for a birth center or home birth, what is your hospital transfer rate? Under what circumstances do you transfer to the hospital?
- Do you have hospital privileges?
- How much fetal monitoring do you do during labor?
- What is your C-section rate?
- How many of your clients deliver their babies without medication?
- How will you help me handle pain?
- How many of your clients are induced? How long past the due date do you allow them to go before scheduling an induction? Do you use natural induction methods?
- If your midwife works in the hospital: Do you use Pitocin to speed up labor? How often? Under what circumstances?
- Right after my baby is born, what is the normal routine? Will I be able to hold my baby immediately?

Birth Goddess: Ina May Gaskin

One of the most famous midwives in the world is the incomparable Ina May Gaskin, whom we personally revere and adore. Her book *Spiritual Midwifery* was the inspiration for our film, *The Business of Being Born*, and we recently made a long-awaited pilgrimage to her beloved midwifery center on The Farm, a historic intentional community in Tennessee. The Farm was founded in 1971, after about 270 young people accompanied Ina May's husband, Stephen Gaskin, on a lecture tour around the country. As the caravan traveled for several months on colorful school buses outfitted as campers, Ina May assisted the birth of several babies even though she had never witnessed a birth before. Eventually, the group pooled their money and bought a thousand acres of wooded land near Summertown, Tennessee, to live in community. The Farm aimed to be as self-sufficient as possible and all the community members took a vow of poverty, grew their own food, and built a school for the children. These young parents-to-be represented a powerful trend to live more closely with nature, and this included a wish to experience birth rather than to be treated as if birth were a medical disaster waiting to happen. At that time, hospitals almost invariably prohibited fathers from being present during the labor and birth of their children, and midwives were almost never employed in hospitals.

The pictures in *Spiritual Midwifery*, which describes many of the births that took place on The Farm, seem right out of the Summer of Love. These "hippie," homespun families look so relaxed and joyous as they are photographed giving birth. The births are described in a celebratory language, replacing painful-sounding words like "contractions" with the more ecstatic "rushes." The state public health officials didn't try to shut the group down or force them into the hospital to have their babies. Instead, officials dropped off a stack of birth and death certificates, and the midwives were able to find two or three physician mentors. Yet The Farm community was as serious about safety as it was passionate about natural birth. Its C-section and intervention rates were way below the national average, and as word of their

(continued)

success spread, women from the surrounding towns began showing up at The Farm to give birth with the midwives.

In the last thirty-five years more than twenty-five hundred babies have been born at The Farm, which has a C-section rate of about 2 percent. And while it is no longer a collective community as it was for the first dozen years, it still is a place where women come from all over the country to have their babies. Several of the original members have built little birth cabins on their property where families can stay when the birth is approaching. (Some have even come from Indonesia and Brazil!) The Farm midwives also attend home births and have a good relationship with the local hospital. Some of the pregnant women we spoke to during our visit were commuting from nearby Alabama, where certified professional midwives are blocked from obtaining legal licensure.

Ina May is a goddess in the birth community for promoting midwifery at a time when it was under attack or illegal in much of the country. She's also revered for the Gaskin maneuver, a technique she learned from a Belize-trained midwife living in Guatemala. This midwife told Ina May that the indigenous midwives she supervised (who were all illiterate) had shown her a better way of resolving the much-feared problem of shoulder dystocia (when the baby's shoulders get stuck in the pelvis) than the way she had been taught in her formal midwifery training. The Gaskin maneuver involves changing the mother's position from sitting or lying back to kneeling on all fours so that the movement of the mother and the wider space between the front and back of her pelvis combine to make birth easier. Sometimes the baby can then be born by the mother's efforts, and if not, the additional space makes it easier for the midwife or doctor to move one of the shoulders around a few degrees, thus freeing the stuck shoulder and saving the baby from an injury to the arm. The Gaskin maneuver is the first obstetrical maneuver named for a midwife and is illustrated in medical textbooks.

5

Doulas

Labor's Love

Actress Kathryn Hahn loved every second of her pregnancy. She and her husband, Ethan, thought of it as a sacred time, almost holy. She was extremely careful about what she ate and took yoga as well as evening walks with her husband when he got home from work. She chose a special pure white cotton nightgown with beautiful lace trim in which she wanted to give birth and she had a doula, Ricki and Abby's friend Ana Paula Markel, whom she trusted completely.

A doula, which is the Greek word for servant, is a fairly recent arrival in maternity, and it's a great one. Our country has sequestered birth off behind the walls and gizmos of the hospital. Few of our friends and family have ever observed a birth or would know how to attend us if we chose them to help, and our loved ones who have given birth probably did so differently, compared to what we are envisioning. Doulas can help you make the decisions you're faced with during childbirth. That's why a growing number of women are hiring them to attend their births.

Doulas are trained through an apprenticeship program during which they take childbirth classes, observe women in labor, and remain after the birth to help in postpartum care. They assist in these births under the guidance of a more experienced doula before they are allowed to assist a midwife or physician on their own. After each of the births, their work is evaluated by a doctor, a midwife, and the parents. Ana Paula has been working as a doula in Los Angeles for twelve years. Kathryn had met Ana Paula at a party two years before she got pregnant. When she found out she was having a baby, Ana Paula was one of the first people she called.

The day before her due date, Kathryn felt a steady trickle of water. Her doctor told her to go to the hospital because, although she wasn't experiencing any signs of labor, if she was losing fluid, she probably needed to be induced. She and Ethan grabbed copies of their birth plan, the iPod with her birth playlist, some family photos, and the white nightgown and stopped for lunch before going to the hospital.

They arrived at the hospital in the middle of a baby boom. The hallway outside the maternity ward was jammed with pregnant women. They waited for two hours in the corridor before they were admitted. As Kathryn's labor hadn't really started, the staff focused on the women who needed immediate attention. They felt like they were in limbo, unable to be admitted but prevented from going home. Ana Paula arrived and could see from the look on Kathryn's face how scared she was that something was going to go horribly wrong.

The room they got was a prelabor room about the size of a closet with no windows, very different from the spacious rooms she and Ethan had seen during their hospital tour. "I had wanted to give him such a beautiful welcome, and we were in a closet!" she said.

Ana Paula brought aromatherapy oil to personalize the room. Ethan put up their family photos and lit candles so that they could make the space their own. Ana Paula had them singing to each other. She taught Ethan how to help Kathryn with her pain and then stepped out of the room to give them some privacy. Initially Ethan had been suspicious of doulas in general, thinking that a stranger would interfere with the intimacy of his experience with his wife. His doubts disappeared when he took birth classes with Ana Paula, and he was even more persuaded that hiring her was a good choice when he saw how she handled their despair.

Ana Paula's calming presence and competence soothed the couple. By the time Ana Paula returned, their mood had transformed and the contractions had started to build. "I couldn't believe we were getting away with this beautiful experience in this setting," Kathryn said. "I would fall asleep and wake up for a contraction. It was like a dream. I had a smile on my face, even though this was in no way what I planned."

This is some of what a doula does in labor support. If you think of childbirth as a journey, the doula can serve as your guide. Many women who hire a doula go through childbirth education with her. She helps you explore your ideas and feelings about birth and can work with you to finalize your birth plan.

She also comes early, sometime in the middle of the first stage of labor, when it's not clear to most first-time moms what should be going on and how fast things should be progressing. The doula is often the first person a woman calls when she goes into labor. And she's with you to the end. The doula will help you manage the pain of early labor by recommending different positions and techniques. She also calls the midwife, if that's who you've chosen to attend your birth, and keeps her informed of your progress. Together they help you decide when is the right moment for the midwife to arrive. Studies show that having a doula around to offer you advice and support can cut your time in labor by two to ten hours and significantly decreases the chance of a C-section.

A woman who trusts her doula and has worked with her over the course of the pregnancy, and through her anxieties about childbirth, may find it easier to surrender to the birth and can find the transition to the second stage of labor more comfortable. Also, a trusted doula who is experienced in birth lessens anxiety by continually reassuring you and your partner that you are doing great and that what you're experiencing is a normal part of birth. Remember how Ricki was freaking out on the stairs at the hospital? She kept thinking that there was something going wrong when in fact nothing was going wrong. That kind of general panic really stalls labor, and it's something a doula is particularly skilled in coaching you through.

Certifying Doulas

Doulas are trained in several programs across the United States. Popular programs include:

Doulas of North America (DONA) requires doulas to attend a sixteen-hour birth doula training course, read five approved books on childbirth, take a twelve-hour childbirth preparation class, complete a breastfeeding workshop, and submit proof that they have attended three births and provide three client evaluations.

Birthworks doulas are childbirth educators. They attend a three-day workshop on childbirth education, facilitate a twenty-hour course on birth, and write about birth, their experiences in birth, and issues related to childbirth in America.

Association of Labor Assistants and Childbirth Educators doulas attend a three-day training class, read three books, audit childbirth education classes, provide written statements, and pass a qualifying exam.

International Childbirth Education Association certifies doulas after they have completed an eighteen-hour workshop and can verify they have practical experience in childbirth and postpartum support.

Doulas don't have a standard fee. We've heard of them charging anywhere from four hundred to three thousand dollars to attend a birth and for prenatal and postpartum visits. This fee is generally not covered by insurance. However, it doesn't hurt to ask your doula to submit a claim and see what happens.

If you're having a hospital birth like Kathryn's, the doula normally meets you at home and helps you manage labor and decide when it is time to go to the hospital. She can help you hold the space for the kind of birth you planned. She will not directly advocate for you, but can remind you and the staff of how you wanted to manage your labor. This doesn't mean she's going to body block the anesthesiologist if you told her previously that you don't want any kind of pain relief. What she can do is slow things down and get you to try to think things over before you agree to something you hadn't planned. She'll try to get you to consider if what the staff is proposing is necessary.

The doula might ask the nurse to step away for a moment if the nurse is about to hook you up to an IV to start Pitocin. At that moment, the doula will remind you that you said in your birth plan you didn't want an augmented labor. She'll describe the effects of Pitocin and how this may increase your chances that you'll end up with an epidural, if this is also something you said you didn't want. In this way the doula is serving as informed consent. Conversely, she might explain that having an epidural might give you the rest you need so you will have the strength to push in the second stage, even if the epidural was not in your birth plan. She's like a well-informed, cool-headed friend standing by who can help you think things through before you agree to them so you don't end up, moment by moment, compromising unwittingly.

As Kathryn and Ethan's birth story demonstrates, the doula can be a service for the partner too. Many times partners become exhausted supporting the mom through a long labor and dealing with the hospital staff. A doula gives your partner breaks, relaxes him, and shows him ways to support you.

If you cannot afford a doula, there are volunteer doulas in some areas (look for these organizations online). Often, but not always, these are less experienced doulas working on their certification.

Kathryn's birth did not go according to plan. Her contractions didn't find a rhythm and she wasn't progressing fast enough for the doctor and the hospital's protocols. She had an epidural and later a C-section. "I had been so on top of it, so powerful, such a warrior," she said. "I was really haunted by how it all came out. As they were prepping me for the C-section, the nurse cut my beautiful nightgown right up the front. That became a symbol to me for all that went wrong." To this day Kathryn wonders if she would have been able to have the birth she'd planned if she had worked with a different doctor or chosen to work with a midwife.

Kathryn and Ethan were incredibly grateful to Ana Paula, however, for helping them have some beautiful memories of a situation that got out of their control and the way she helped them come to terms with it afterwards. "She helped me to embrace the birth I had and stop dwelling on the birth I wanted," Kathryn said.

Red Flag—Doula

Ask the doula you're thinking of hiring for your birth how many clients she takes in an average month. If it's anything higher than five, this is a red flag. She's overscheduled.

You can find a doula through referrals from friends and family or your caregiver. You can also find one online. Women we interviewed for this book who had births that disappointed them and that were marred by what they see as unnecessary interventions recommend that you find the doula first and ask her to recommend an obstetrician or midwife. Doulas know many of the doctors practicing in your area and, once you've decided what kind of birth you want, can give you a list of doctors and midwives who support your ideas. Also, as we mentioned in the section on hospitals, make sure to check that your hospital will allow your doula to attend you at birth and establish if the hospital will allow the doula to be present all the way through the birth.

This is a very intimate service you're hiring someone to perform, so chemistry between the two of you is key. You want to feel relaxed with your doula, comfortable, and secure. Even if she comes highly recommended, if you don't click with her, move on. Some very progressive hospitals have doulas on staff, but that's another thing altogether. Although it's a great idea, this would not be a doula you've been working with for your entire pregnancy and therefore not someone with whom you have a close relationship. But what do we know? According to the first birth that Ana Paula handled on her own, sometimes all a couple needs is someone to tell them that they're doing just fine.

Picking a Doula for Youla

Nickie Tilsner, a doula and doula trainer in the San Francisco Bay Area, advises moms-to-be on how to choose a doula. She recommends that you pay careful attention to how your energy matches hers. "Experience is not the key here," Nickie said. "You may feel completely comfortable with someone who has just completed her training. And you might feel uncomfortable with the diva doula who has all the clients in the community, or vice versa."

Your idea of what constitutes a good birth should match too, but more important than that is to find someone who is flexible.

"You never know how your labor is going to go, and you want someone who can go with you," Nickie said. "I believe that it's the best thing for the baby to not have any medication at birth, but I also believe that babies feel what their moms feel emotionally. I don't want babies to be imprinted by the suffering of their mothers at birth. If an epidural is the one thing that can give a mom the relief or relaxation that she may need to enjoy her birth and even prevent a C-section, I would definitely opt for medication. You need that kind of flexibility."

The first birth Ana Paula worked on her own was with an Israeli couple who didn't speak much English. Her job was to supervise the birth and call the midwife when it was getting close to the second stage. The couple was very connected and intuitive about birth. The husband wanted to massage his wife's back. As Ana Paula couldn't speak Hebrew, she simply gave him the thumbs-up and a big smile. Then he wanted to take his wife into the shower. Another smiling thumbs-up from Ana Paula. When they were in the shower, he started to give his wife counter-pressure for back labor. Ana Paula moved his hands lower on his wife's back to a more effective position and gave another thumbs-up.

The birth went flawlessly. Ana Paula thought she wouldn't get a very good review because she didn't do much, in her opinion. The couple raved about what a great job she did. "That taught me a lesson," she said. "People only need a little bit of encouragement. They want someone to tell them they are doing it right. Most of the time, you just smile and leave them alone."

Questions for Your Doula

Questions for birth doulas are generally along the lines of:

- How many births have you witnessed?
- Are you certified? By whom? For how long?
- Why did you choose to be a doula?
- Do you have a backup that I can meet?
- How many clients do you take a month?
- When do you join me in labor?
- How long do you stay after my baby is born?
- What is your "philosophy" about birth?
- How do you feel about working with couples who choose epidurals and other interventions?
- How does your payment schedule work? Do you have a sliding scale?
- What happens if we end up needing a cesarean?

Chapter

6

The Guest List

Birth as a Private Party

One freaky thing about having a baby is how much other people see your pregnancy as a chance to give you unsolicited advice. It seems like everyone is an expert on pregnancy, even people who haven't had babies. The bigger you get, the larger the circle of people who want to tell you what you should be doing. Strangers, people who normally wouldn't give you a second look, are drawn to that big belly. They touch you! They don't even ask permission. And then they start going on about their birth, or their sister's, or their great aunt's. Even if you want to haul off and smack them, you don't. You know they mean well and you don't want to seem like the pregnancy bitch instead of the birth goddess.

Maybe it would be better for all concerned if you did smack them. It's good preparation for how you're going to be, or how you should feel free to be, once you are in labor.

Everyone may believe they are experts in pregnancy, but you are the world's biggest expert on you. You are the only person truly qualified to say who should be around you at the moment of this birth, and at that time you should be able to say and do whatever you feel like without trying to be good or nice or worrying about other people's feelings. Only people whom you trust completely, who approve of your birth plan, and who you don't mind seeing you naked should be present at the birth.

Well, that certainly shortens the list. Particularly the naked part.

The time we live in is an interesting moment in the history of birth. For centuries birth was something that women kept inside a protected circle. No men allowed. As the medical model of birth took over from the womanly rituals, women were walled off in the hospital, separated from their families, and male doctors took over the birth chamber. When women started agitating for a different kind of hospital birth in the seventies, hospitals began to allow their partners in. Now some allow partners, doulas, and other supporters in too.

It's one of those times when they tell you that "you have a lot of choices" and you think, "Please can I have fewer?" It's a time to set boundaries lest you regret including some people, depending on how things evolve. At the end of Jorie Walker's regrettable hospital birth, she had a small vaginal tear, so she lay there, feet in the stirrups, fully exposed, waiting for someone to come stitch her up. She had to wait an hour. It took the staff twenty minutes just to drape her. "And my father was in the room the entire time," she said.

If Your Partner Is Freaking Out about Your Birth Plan

Let's say you want something other than the standard hospital birth and your partner does not. Some doulas, midwives, and childbirth educators see this as a bad sign in your relationship, but we're going to call it an opportunity for personal growth. That's the way we think of birth for you, so why not for your partner too?

Most of the time the reason people are phobic about a birth center or a midwife or a home birth is because they don't know too much about them. As these birth choices are unconventional, your partner might even suspect you've lost a bit of your mind in pregnancy and are choosing something that might damage your baby. Compassion here. You may have walked this path yourself before you decided how you wanted to give birth, and you need to show your partner how you came to your decision.

Not to promote ourselves too much here, but the easiest way to start the conversation is to show your partner our movie, *The Business of Being Born*. It covers all the territory plus it is a good preview of birth and might even get your partner fired up about the politics of birth. Plus, no reading. We know how a lot of guys are about reading. If he gets really into it, there are books tailored to the partners such as the Bradley Method's *Natural Childbirth the Bradley Way*. Even if you don't want to follow the Bradley Method, this is a book that really focuses on the importance of the partner while conveying much useful information. There's also Penny Simkin's *The Birth Partner: A Complete Guide to Childbirth for Dads, Doulas, and All Other Labor Companions*.

If you're considering a birth center or a midwife, talk to them about your partner's feelings. Most of them have faced this kind of situation before. Many have in their files contact information for husbands and other lovers who dragged their feet at first but were ecstatic with the end result. They may be willing to put your partner in touch with one of those people who can take them step-by-step through what they feared and where they ended, which can be extremely persuasive.

In the end, though, it's your baby and your body. Maybe it sounds mean and exclusionary, but you are the birth goddess. In this instance, you've also got a bit of the birth bitch. You have to birth this baby the way it feels right to you and your body, and if other people get their feelings bruised, well, you'll see them on the other side. And you'll be happy for all the help they can give you with the baby.

Birth is not a party, like a wedding, where you have to worry about offending those who were not invited. Let's review that list of qualifications again: You should only invite people you trust, who approve of your birth plan, and who you don't mind seeing you naked.

You might not ever get completely naked. Ricki was. She walked all around her apartment as naked as a baby while she was laboring with Owen and everybody around her just had to deal with it. Even if you are horrified by the idea of doing that, know that you are going to be naked in some way or another. You're going to be moaning or swearing or crying or telling people to piss off and probably announcing at some point near transition that somebody needs to "just get this ****ing baby out." This is something you *need to do*. Being raw like that, completely open, helps move that baby along. You're also going to be radiant, powerful, at your most vulnerable, and at your strongest. The full range of you will be on display in the course of this labor. This is not something that everyone can handle. So you want to have as your birth partners people with whom you can be completely uninhibited. This can be as many people as you feel comfortable having around or as few as you think are necessary for you to be fully supported.

Which brings us to your mother.

How have things been going with mom?

Pregnancy is a huge sign that you are your own woman and you are going to do things your way. Some moms don't handle this very well. Who are we kidding? Some daughters don't do too well either. Of all the people who give you random advice during pregnancy, your mom's comes with the most consequences. Remember how Jill Williams's mom wouldn't speak to her when she sent her the e-mail message that she was having a home birth for her third child? Unlike strangers on the street, if Mom tells you to do something or not do something, she's definitely going to follow up to see if you did what you were told like a good little girl.

Maybe your mom gives the greatest advice in the world, or at least knows how to keep her mouth shut when she senses you've decided definitively about something. Even if you have a really strong relationship with your mom and call her every day to tell her everything, you still don't have to have her at the birth. San Francisco Bay Area midwife Tekoa King advises her clients who don't want Mom around to tell her, "Mom, I'm going to be in a lot of pain and I may be saying things and acting in ways that make you really uncomfortable. If you're there, you'll want to be my mom because I'm still your little girl. You might want to try to make the pain go away and I just can't have you trying to do that." By counseling her like that, you honor and respect her but still create a boundary that most likely she won't try to cross.

This is not just about personal preferences. Having the right people can help your labor go more smoothly and having the wrong people can stall your labor. Midwives know from watching many women in labor that the presence of a negative or critical individual can make the mom inhibited and less able to yield to her contractions, and that having a loving team of supporters can encourage the whole body to relax through the phases of labor.

When you go into labor, you're primal. Your intellect isn't much use to you. As a result, the walls between the compartments where you store your traumas and resentments can come tumbling down because you don't have your inhibitions in place to keep them solid. If you have major issues with your mother or with your partner or doubts about becoming a mother, all of these can come up during labor and bring the process to a halt.

We're just assuming that you're going to want your partner there. Most women these days do. Maybe we shouldn't assume anything about that. Kathy Herron and other midwives and doulas all have stories of how emotional issues stall labor, and in each case they cite, it's clear that part of preparing for labor is ensuring that these fears and conflicts are addressed before the woman surrenders to her primal self in labor. In some cases, the hesitation is because the woman wants a specific person to be in the room and that person hasn't arrived.

Preparing Your Partner for Birth

Going through pregnancy and birth together can be a great opportunity to build a new dimension in your relationship with your partner. You've got to depend on him and, if you are on the same page and he comes through for you, it can be the best preparation possible for becoming a family. That said, if he's disengaged or overwhelmed, it could be difficult for you. Use the pregnancy as an opportunity to deepen your communication with each other.

The best preparation for birth is to take a good childbirth class together. The teacher will describe pregnancy and birth and, in a good class, also

(continued)

describe the different interventions and pain relief options. This will give you two much to talk about in deciding the kind of birth you want.

Prior to the birth, it's important to figure out how your partner can support you in labor. What will you want him to do? And of those things, what do you think your partner is capable of doing? The following questions can help you think about your partner's role on the big day.

Have you talked over your thoughts and feelings about the coming child and your fears about birth? This is a good starting place. If you explore these things thoroughly, it shows how you can communicate with each other during birth. While you may be frightened about the birth, he can be too.

How does your partner act when you are in pain? Does he want to rush to rescue you? Does he feel guilty because he can't protect you? He may need careful coaching to know how to comfort and encourage you when things get tough.

Are things between you and your partner in a good place right now? Are you having trust issues? Was this a wanted child? Are there infidelity problems? If there are any issues simmering between you, seek help to resolve them before the birth so they will not affect you on that day.

Have you agreed on a birth plan? You need to be a team during birth. Part of being a team is having a shared idea of how to handle the surprising twists and turns of birth. He may need to be your defender at times when the hospital or birth center staff wants to deviate from that plan. If he's got to oppose authority, you want him to be unconflicted, and part of that is having a plan you both agree on. It's vitally important that he be supportive of your doctor, midwife, and/or doula.

Is the pattern in your relationship that you take care of him? You're not going to be able to take care of anyone but yourself while

you are in labor. You may be angry and rude to him and he's just going to have to get over it. Warn him about this. If he's pouting when you need him, things will just get worse.

Do you think he can give you what you need while you are in labor? Maybe he's not so good at massage. Maybe he's the kind of guy who makes dumb jokes when you bring up something personal or emotional. These are also things that should be talked about before the birth.

Are your expectations of support realistic? He's not going to be somebody else. He's going to be your partner under stress. Have a realistic expectation for what he can provide and if there are things outside his skills that you think you'll need, have someone else who can provide them present at the birth.

When Abby was shooting our documentary she witnessed a hospital birth where the baby's father didn't show up and the mom never dilated past six centimeters. She seemed completely disengaged from the process. She never asked for any pain medication, but then she didn't seem to be feeling anything. She was lying in bed watching television while her mother sat at her side complaining about what a mess she'd made of her life and how the father was never going to show up. The mom wasn't interested in moving around and eventually after hours of this she had a C-section. It's hard to say if the dad's showing up would have had any effect on this situation, but for some women the presence or absence of their partner is the one thing they really need.

One of midwife Kathy Herron's clients was a woman who was having a very easy labor with her third baby. The labor was nearly complete; Kathy could see the baby's head crowning and thought that with one or two more pushes the baby would be out. Kathy put on her gloves to catch the baby when suddenly the contractions stopped and the baby's hair was no longer visible. It had retracted into the birth canal! When Kathy asked her what was going on, the mom said she couldn't deliver the baby unless her husband was in the room. Kathy left to retrieve him from the waiting room.

Kathy came upon the husband pacing in the waiting room. He told her he was worried that he would throw up or pass out if he witnessed the baby being born. Kathy explained his wife's situation, but he refused to enter the birthing suite. "We've got to work something out because she is not going to have the baby without you," she said. Kathy led him to the door to the room and put a screen in the doorway so the husband couldn't see anything. From that distance, he called to his wife. "I'm here. I'm right here honey. I love you more than anything," he said, "you can do it." With the sound of his words, the mom started to push again and Kathy again saw the top of the baby's head. "Should I put my gloves back on?" she asked the mom. She'd barely gotten her gloves on when the mom pushed the baby right out.

Chapter

7

For Sexual Abuse Survivors,
a Healing

One of the reasons you have to protect yourself so well during labor and pick those who will surround you carefully is that in labor so much of you is exposed. Old traumas from the past can come rushing forward. In that balancing act between surrender and control, those who previously have been victimized by sexual abuse can be profoundly affected by the process of labor.

This can be uncomfortable to talk about, but then many things surrounding childbirth are. One of the rarely discussed aspects of childbirth is that it can actually be a sexual experience. Sorry if your eyes are bugging out right now at the very suggestion that such a dramatic and painful experience has a sexual side to it. At first we thought of it as shocking too. But think of it logically: the movement of something through the vagina coupled with the fact that one of the things that can encourage contractions to progress is having your partner stimulate your nipples. (Sexual stimulation increases the production of oxytocin, the hormone that promotes stronger, longer contractions.) For this reason women who have been sexually abused sometimes have a difficult time with labor.

Experts estimate that more than a quarter of women have been sexually abused, and some estimate as much as 40 percent. Some women have shoved this memory aside in order to get on with their lives and others have faced the experience in therapy and believe they have put it behind them. "Even if they have addressed it in therapy, childbirth can bring that memory back. For many abuse survivors, not all, pregnancy and childbirth represents the biggest challenge they have for healing," said birth counselor Penny Simkin, who has written about, taught, and counseled many survivors and their caregivers. "If they have worked on and resolved their abuse issues, they often are shocked that they are coming up again."

Some women who have been abused as children are frightened by the lack of control labor represents. They may not trust their bodies and see them as a source of shame. They also can feel very uncomfortable around authority figures. As a result, they are more likely to feel as though they are not being understood or listened to by their caregivers.

Having their privacy violated by childbirth is traumatic, and the fingers or instruments that the medical staff insert as part of the routine vaginal exams and the monitoring of labor can have a double meaning for them. In *When Survivors Give Birth: Understanding and Healing the Effects of Early Sexual Abuse on Childbearing Women*, Penny Simkin and psychotherapist Phyllis Klaus note some of the commonplace instructions caregivers say to laboring women such as, "Open your legs," "Relax your bottom," and "Relax and it won't hurt so much." As the authors point out, "In the eyes of the survivor, control is seen as the antithesis of victimization." In labor though, attempts at control prevent a mother from releasing the baby.

Women who have been sexually abused may have major concerns about modesty during birth. Others may be fearful of forceps or vacuum extraction and other large objects' being inserted into their vaginas. Heightened fears of this kind should be a clue to your caregiver that you need some special treatment to give birth safely. The book notes the case of a woman who was pregnant for the first time and was certain that she would be unable to let go enough to deliver vaginally. She told the nurse that she'd suffered constipation all her life and every bowel movement or urination was a strain for her. As she and the nurse talked, she revealed that she feared her vagina was too mutilated to deliver a baby and she just might be ripped apart.

She listed her concerns during labor as fear of pain, fear that the birth would remind her of her childhood abuse, and fear that she would be ripped apart either by the birth or by a cesarean. She also was very concerned about modesty.

The nurse planned to answer her concerns by having only the people who truly supported her around her and asking others to step outside the room when she needed to be examined during labor. The nurse pledged that only one person would do her vaginal exams and would proceed at the woman's pace. The nurse also told her that she would be carefully coached to use positions while pushing that would protect her modesty and allow her pushing to be most effective. The nurse also pledged that the woman would be fully informed, counseled, and reassured if a cesarean became necessary.

Melissa Uses Birth to Come into Her Own

Melissa doesn't know exactly how old she was when her uncle started sexually abusing her. She can guess what era it was because she remembers what house her family lived in then and that for a long time no one in her family believed her when she told the story. Much later, when she had become a promiscuous teenager, she used her body in a way she thought men did: to get pleasure and flee from her feelings. All the adults in the family thought she was a tramp who couldn't be trusted to tell the truth about her sex life.

When she moved to Los Angeles, her self-abuse escalated. As she closed in on thirty, she made a list of the things she wanted to accomplish before her birthday and on that list was to get an AIDS test. "What's wrong with this picture?" she asked herself. She began attending an incest survivors support group to deal with the abuse. Luckily she met the man who would become her husband shortly after that, and by the time she turned thirty-three she was married and pregnant.

The pregnancy went fine, but the idea of labor scared her. Like many

(continued)

women, she feared turning into her mother, particularly while giving birth. Her mother told her that when she was giving birth to Melissa, she had been drugged heavily and let her husband make all the decisions. She said she wished she'd been more aware. From that moment Melissa decided she wanted to do everything the exact opposite of the way her mother had. She would be fully aware, completely in charge of the decisions, and would not take any drugs at all.

"The idea of various doctors coming in and hovering about horrified me," Melissa said. "I had that fear of being disconnected and not being respected as a woman. I was worried about my body getting ruined. The scar from a C-section was not on my list of things I wanted."

She sought out Los Angeles obstetrician Dr. Paul Crane, "warm and loving without being inappropriate, willing to let me make my decisions," and doula Ana Paula Markel, who had worked with sexual abuse survivors before. "I wanted to know that she had my back and she did, literally," Melissa said. "She held my back when I was in labor."

When her water broke in the hospital, Melissa was repulsed. "I'm a person who doesn't even like to blow her nose in front of other people! But Ana Paula cleaned it right up." Dr. Crane helped her take positions that helped the baby move when her squats weren't being as effective as she thought they would be. When she pushed her daughter out, it was like she gave birth to a new self, she said. Melissa was so in awe of the way she had controlled the experience, not been a victim of it, and had created this beautiful new life.

"I didn't feel like a victim anymore," she said of the birth of her girl. "I had been told I was weak and passive and promiscuous, but really I was none of those things. I felt like I had overcome who I was told I was supposed to be. My true self came out. It was better than therapy."

Although many caregivers ask about a history of sexual abuse as part of the general background questions, some women are too ashamed to tell them or have shut the experience out of their minds. Experienced caregivers can often tell that a woman may have a history of abuse even if she does not recall it or chooses not to acknowledge it. An inability to tolerate vaginal exams is frequently a clue. When a kind, experienced caregiver sees this reaction, she proceeds gently and slowly. When Penny works with a survivor who has issues with vaginal exams, she wants the woman "to know that this is not abnormal. When women have such difficulties there are good reasons, and they are not sissies or weaklings," she said. "It takes a lot of courage to talk to her care provider about her abuse, especially since many care providers are not that sensitive. If she doesn't get a good response then she should ideally leave that care provider and go to a better one. That is not always possible, and if not, she should try to state her needs in a letter to the staff and recruit the aid of her partner or an understanding advocate, like a doula or confident friend."

For some survivors of sexual abuse, like Ricki, having a good birth experience can be part of healing from that terrible experience from the past. "It is wonderful when an abuse survivor has reached the point when with her own inner strength she can push the pain out once and for all. Unfortunately, not everyone is at this level of readiness, and birth can result in retraumatization if she receives insensitive care," Simkin said. "Birth can be healing when she feels empowered because people have listened to her and are committed to making this the best birth experience possible, as the woman defines it, and protect her at all costs."

Ricki: Birth as Healing

When I was six or seven my parents hired someone to do work around the house. He sexually abused me. I never talked about it until I was in my early twenties. It was my secret. I always questioned why I wasn't promiscuous and why I was very overweight. I didn't want to be attractive. I kept thinking, "Is that the reason?" So I kept just putting two and two together. That's what I was dealing with, my hidden thing.

And then, I think, I worked it out in therapy, I got to a point where I felt like it was common. I do think abuse can inhibit you from having a positive birthing experience. It didn't stop me, though.

I think the birthing process, even my first birth, felt like a miracle, like my

(continued)

body was just the most amazing thing. But I don't think I fully accepted my body until my second birth, when Owen was born. Then I totally looked at my body in amazement, like look what I'm capable of. It is amazing that we can carry children and give birth.

After Owen was born, I started to lose weight easily. Well, it definitely didn't fall off. I made a decision, but it was the easiest time I'd ever tried. I kept losing four pounds, losing five pounds, losing all this weight so quickly. I don't know how to explain it other than it just felt like this purging of that pain and trauma from the past.

INTERVENTIONS
The Slippery Slope

As we've discussed, modern medicine has amazing ways to identify and help mothers and babies in distress. Technology and techniques developed in the last forty years support babies who otherwise would have died and mothers who might have hemorrhaged to death. When doctors intervene wisely to save the life of a mom or a baby, they are skilled providers doing what they do best, and everyone owes them huge gratitude. Yet those who operate under the medical model of childbirth can feel as though they aren't doing their job unless they use their tools to intervene. As a result, women often find themselves agreeing to one drug, which their doctor tells them will make labor go more smoothly or safely, and then slipping quickly toward a C-section.

Critics of the way babies are born in this country call this the cascade of interventions. Cascade is such a happy word that it almost seems out of place in this context because it reminds you of coasting happily down a frothy waterfall. The way it applies to childbirth is the loss of control over aspects of birth that you wanted to manage. The Pitocin that helps you get your labor started on what your doctor says is the right schedule—almost half of the women in the Listening to Mothers II survey reported that their doctors wanted to induce them—makes the contractions so much stronger that you need pain relief. So then you're on an epidural. Seventy-six percent of women in that survey, which included vaginal and cesarean births, received epidurals.

Part of the cascade effect is that many times no one tells you about the downsides of interventions. Things happen pretty quickly in the hospital and informed consent isn't always the staff's highest priority, even if getting you to sign the release form is. If you don't know the risks, how are you supposed to weigh them against the benefits? In this section, we're going to speak candidly about different kinds of interventions so that now, as you sit calmly reading a book and are not in labor, you can think these things through and talk them over with your partner and your caregiver. That way, if you find yourself in a situation where things are moving quickly and there is pressure for you to decide, you can say, "Wait! There is a reason I decided against this. Everybody, let's just slow down and give me a minute to think this over."

First off, no matter what they tell you, every drug you take affects your baby. Even the wonder drug of the epidural, which is only supposed to block the transmission of pain to the brain, affects the baby. Every decision you make about taking drugs while in labor has to have that among the considerations. Plus, you shouldn't believe everything you hear about drugs and procedures that are supposed to be for the benefit of your baby or the ease of your labor and birth. Many women have unwittingly consented to drugs and interventions that were poorly tested and led to tragic results.

The most well-known one is thalidomide, a drug that women took because their doctors told them back in the 1950s and early 1960s it would ease morning sickness and could help them get to sleep. The drug had not been tested on pregnant women. When they took it, their baby's long limb bones stopped forming. Ten thousand babies were born with their hands perched on their shoulders or feet right up against their hip bones. You've probably seen pictures of these children. Can you imagine how angry their mothers felt for being part of an experiment in drug use? This terrible tragedy led to a federal Food and Drug Administration rule that drugs that were specifically prescribed to be used on pregnant women should first be tested on pregnant women. All we can say to that is: Duh!

Problem solved, right? Not exactly. In the present day there is Cytotec, a drug originally developed in the 1980s to treat stomach ulcers and now more commonly called by its generic name, misoprostol. Prominently on the drug label the manufacturer warned that it was not to be used by pregnant women because its big side effect is severe uterine contractions. Instead of heeding that warning, shortly after it was introduced for ulcers hospitals all over the country started using it to induce labor. Cytotec, unlike the Pitocin drip, cannot be easily dialed down or scaled back. Cytotec is also cheaper than Pitocin.

Dr. Marsden Wagner, who wrote about this extensively in his book *Born in the USA*, estimates that in the ten years before the Association of Obstetricians and Gynecologists recommended against using Cytotec, doctors prescribed it for twenty-five thousand women who were trying for a VBAC. Approximately a thousand women's uteruses ruptured. Dr. Wagner calculates that between fifty and two hundred babies died as a result of this as did between ten and twenty women. In 2008 the FDA clarified its position on misoprostol: They still do not recommend it but advised doctors that if they were going to use it on pregnant women, the women needed to be fully informed of the increased risks it presents for uterine rupture and maternal death.

"There are a lot of doctors who will say the FDA has approved it," Dr. Wagner said when we spoke with him. "One of the terrible problems is that in using drugs on pregnant women, it's safe until it's proven dangerous. That is the antiprecautionary approach." Despite the fact that the Physicians' Desk Reference says Cytotec is not recommended for pregnant women, many medical professionals attest that it works well when administered correctly but should never be given to women who are having a VBAC. Today, many doctors and midwives feel confident that Cytotec can be used safely and effectively, but only in the appropriate circumstances.

Stories like these, while by far rare occurrences, are worrying. They remind us how much is at stake here and that every attempt to interfere or interrupt the natural process of birth has to be considered very carefully. Even though your baby is strong and resilient, a little super hero making the journey down the birth canal, every intervention, every drug, carries with it some risks. You need to know those risks. We'll start talking about drugs by talking about the epidural, which is by far the most commonly prescribed method of pain relief during labor.

8

Epidurals

You Haven't Got Time for the Pain

During labor in most hospitals, the staff hawk epidurals like sodas at the ballpark. Nurses and doctors keep coming into the room every half hour or so to ask you if you want an epidural. Get your epidurals right here! In any size you need them, right here but going fast! Why is it that during the entire course of pregnancy everyone's jumping all over you if you have so much as a wine cooler, but suddenly when you are in labor, the front door has blown off the pharmacy cabinet and they're offering you narcotics and opium derivatives and stuff that, chemically speaking, looks a lot like cocaine?

When caregivers are pushing epidurals, they keep telling you that it's a great thing because it blocks the transmission of the pain to the brain but it doesn't affect the baby. You can get the best of all worlds: no pain, clear head, and no groggy baby. Who could turn that down? Few women do. By some estimates, 80 percent of women have their babies with the aid of an epidural.

But guess what? It does get to the baby. It's not like the anesthesiologist actually inserts a temporary dam between the lower half of the body and the upper half of the body to block the sensations. She injects narcotics into a tiny space where the nerves exit the spinal cord.

The difference between a shot of Demerol and an epidural is that with an epidural, the narcotics are specifically targeted to disengage just the lower half. So unlike getting a shot of Demerol, a commonly used painkiller similar to morphine in its effect, where you'd be drugged out, nauseous, passed out, and uncommunicative, epidural mom can sit and chat. Every once in a while she can look over and see if the monitor says she's still having contractions.

There's a critical moment right around the time that you're five centimeters dilated when the epidural is the most effective and safest to administer, but recently anesthesiologists have broadened their idea of when a woman can get one. Previously they didn't want to give it too early because they believed that an epidural slowed the progress of labor. Getting one too early might mean that you'd take forever to dilate. At eight or nine centimeters, the caregivers used to advise against getting one because the lack of sensation can make it difficult to push. If you were that far along, they would advise you to just tough it out. Now that the approach to use has changed, you can get one the moment you're admitted to the hospital if you want one.

If you're not steady and in the right position, the drug might go where it's not supposed to go. The anesthesiologist could damage your nerves or paralyze you. In some cases, the epidural, when handled ineptly, only numbs half of the lowest regions of your body, which doesn't do you a whole lot of good in labor.

To begin, the anesthesiologist tells you to sit up with your back arched like a cat so he can get full access to your back. Then you're numbed with a little Novocain. It's good that you are facing away because you might freak if you saw the size of the needle he's about to stick in you.

He threads this hollow needle into a tiny space between the vertebrae at the lower part of your spine and pierces the intraspinal ligaments. He tries to get this needle in when you're between contractions so you don't screw up his aim. Everybody's spine is slightly different. Depending on your spine and the skill of the anesthesiologist, this procedure takes from five to ten minutes or as much as thirty if the woman is significantly overweight. In the end of the second stage of labor, when powerful contractions are coming very close together, it might be hard for you to hold still long enough for the anesthesiologist to get the needle in the right spot. Contractions also tighten up your back. A relaxed back makes a much better target for this delicate procedure.

When he hits it just right, he sticks a tube through the needle, takes the needle out, and shoots in a test dose of the drugs to make sure he's in the correct spot. After that, pain is no longer able to make its way up to your brain. The tube remains in place to allow for continuous delivery of the drugs, which are usually an analgesic or an anesthetic. Half an hour to ninety minutes later, the pain is blocked.

The epidural differs from a spinal block, a less common method of dealing with labor pain, in two ways. A spinal block is a single shot aimed directly into the spinal fluid that bathes the outside of the cord with pain killers and works for just a few hours. The spine is a closed system so in order to inject the drug, the doctor has to take out the same amount of spinal fluid as he's about to inject. An advantage of the epidural is that it allows doctors to increase or decrease the dosage as labor progresses. Anesthesiologists also have a combo-platter option that includes the spinal to eliminate the pain before attaching the epidural.

Once the epidural is in, you're gliding down the cascade. You have to be closely monitored. The staff turns you from side to side to make sure the drug is distributed equally in both sides of your pelvis; it's pretty common that the epidural is only partially effective on one side of your body. If the baby is in distress with you on one side, they will rock you to the other side for better blood perfusion.

In close to a fifth of women, epidurals cause a big drop in blood pressure, which can cut off oxygen to your baby. So along with the epidural catheter, you get an IV, an electronic fetal heart rate monitor, and a blood pressure cuff that inflates on its own to record your vital signs. You also get a catheter in your bladder to drain away urine because you're immobilized and too numb to know when to pee. They might call it a walking epidural if the dosage is kept to a minimum, but being hooked up to all these devices and drainage tubes makes it pretty hard to walk. But, as Ricki did with Milo, you still have enough feeling in your legs to squat with the aid of the bar.

The advantage of this kind of drug is that most women have their pain completely eliminated, which can be particularly helpful if you are wiped out from the effort of a long labor and need a rest. The effort required and the feeling of disappointment that labor has not progressed can leave the mom in a terrible state: exhausted but with a big dose of adrenaline in her veins from the effort of labor. Remember that adrenaline stalls labor because when it increases, oxytocin (the hormone that causes contractions) decreases. Having an epidural in a situation like that can give the mom a break and normalize labor for her. Because there are disadvantages and risks with an epidural, women not in that situation should think clearly and carefully about having one.

Okay, now the super-scary side effects, which thankfully are pretty rare. Women who get epidurals have a three times higher chance of dying than those who don't, but overall that's still a small number. In one out of five hundred epidurals the woman is temporarily paralyzed and in one out of half a million cases, that paralysis is permanent. There's also a bunch of side effects: backaches (which in rare cases last more than a year), infection in the injection site, an itchy incision, nausea, shivering, and headaches that linger for days or in some cases a week or more after the birth. Headaches, which come from spinal fluid leaking out from the place where the epidural used to be, are pretty common. One out of one hundred women who have epidurals get them, and to cure the pain she has to go back to the doctor and have him take a bit of her blood to make a clot that is used to patch the leak.

Keep in mind that, for most everyone, having an epidural slows labor down. Without one, the muscles of the pelvic floor are strong and resilient. They help your baby move into the right position to descend. After you've had an epidural, these muscles are slack. The perfect epidural would dull the pain but not the sensation. If it's a less-than-perfect one, you're numb everywhere south of the waist and you don't know when to push, so you have to be coached by the nurse watching your contractions on the monitor. This means you're not sure how hard and how effectively you are pushing. Immobilized in bed, there is a limited number of positions you can take to help the baby progress.

Every woman has a right to pain medication in childbirth if she wants it, and no one should feel guilty or less of a mother for requesting pain relief. But one thing to consider is that once you are numb from the waist down, you are protected from the über-pain of crashing Pitocin-fueled contractions but your baby is not. So when you are numb from the waist down and your baby is being pounded by mega-contractions, you are dependent on machines and monitors to watch out for that baby. You are no longer in control of your labor and now need to be instructed and told when to push. This changes the dynamic again of your taking total control.

These effects combined may explain why women who have epidurals have a higher risk of having a C-section or having their baby pulled out with forceps or by a vacuum extraction. Delivery by forceps or vacuum increases the number of vaginal tears and episiotomies. About a fifth of women who get epidurals get a fever during labor, which can be tough on the baby and affects postpartum care. When the staff sees that the baby has a fever, they have to check for a uterine infection when the baby emerges. If your baby has a fever, your baby and you will be separated during those crucial first minutes.

In order to prevent these things, you might ask that they let the epidural wear off during the pushing phase so that you can get some sensation and control. Some women can't tolerate this because getting an epidural cuts off their bodies' production of natural painkilling endorphins, which increase gradually to handle the increasing sensations as labor progresses. When the staff turns off the epidural, there's no defense against the sudden spike in pain.

Babies whose mothers have had epidurals can experience problems too. The biggest ones, as we mentioned earlier, are the risks that oxygen will get cut off and the elevated heart rate and fever. Some lactation consultants can tell quickly which babies have been involved in an epidural birth because they frequently have trouble latching onto the breast. Some midwives can tell at a glance which babies have been exposed to epidurals because they're more sluggish and can be hard to soothe.

9

Inductions and Pitocin
Let's Get This Party Started

Inducing your labor, meaning employing some external means to get labor started, has become so widespread and uncontroversial that, when Abby called some New York obstetricians during the research for our film, their voice mail had among its choices, "If you're calling to schedule your induction, please press two."

There are valid medical reasons for induction, which apply to about 10 percent of pregnancies. Doctors induce about 40 percent of women, with the most common reason being that the caregiver says they are "overdue." This means many more women are being induced than are medically necessary.

Much of this is because of perceived liability and lack of trust in the birth process, or to stop the irritation of the mom who is so sick of being pregnant she could scream. The pregnant mom and everyone around her get so fixated on the due date that this impatience starts to build weeks before the doctor has told her that her baby is due to be born. Many obstetrical practices routinely offer induction as a delivery option after you've reached thirty-eight weeks.

When people find out you're pregnant, they always ask when the baby

Overdue: Why Your Baby Is Not
Like a Library Book

Establishing a due date for a pregnancy is a routine part of your first prenatal visit but it's essentially a guess. The doctor takes out that little wheel, spins it to the date of your last period, and then reads the dial and gives you a due date. Even though this is all done with averages, the due date becomes a huge determining factor in whether you are a candidate for induction. Not everyone ovulates the same way so this initial calculation could be as much as a week off of the reality of your cycle.

The assumption that pregnancy lasts forty weeks is something the doctors pulled out of the history books. A German obstetrician back in the 1800s declared that pregnancy takes forty weeks and we haven't budged from that idea since. More recent studies of healthy women show that first-time mothers typically go a week or more past that. Modern obstetrics starts talking about inducing at forty-one weeks even though for most women that's just at the moment when their pregnancy is complete and their baby is getting ready for labor. In fact, in France doctors say pregnancy lasts forty-one weeks and plot due dates accordingly. Hey, that's France where we guess everything is more leisurely.

But wait, we've got ultrasounds to help determine when the baby is ready. While those pictures are extremely satisfying, they're not a very good way to establish the due date. They can be off by as much as five days in the first trimester and even more at the end of pregnancy. Five days is a pretty big margin of error where your due date is concerned. (However, it depends on when in the first trimester the ultrasound is done. Ask that it be done at six or seven weeks, when it has a margin of error of only three days.)

As an alternative, Dr. Stuart Fischbein suggests a due "window." This alleviates the problem of Aunt Mary writing down a due date and calling every day to ask, "Why isn't your doctor doing something?" He uses a window from three weeks before the calculated date to two weeks after. This is essentially a five-week window, so when friends ask when you're due, you just say somewhere between May 1 and June 4, for example.

is due. You repeat that date so often that it becomes fixed in your mind like a goal, a cutoff point. The bigger you get, the more often that date comes up. On that day, the phone vibrates in your pocket all day long with people asking if you are in labor. You begin to feel like you and your baby are disappointing everyone by not performing according to the schedule. You've missed a crucial deadline. Doctors ought to tell you that the due date is pretty random. Yet from the moment you pass the due date, many doctors start eyeing the calendar and begin to think about inducing you.

An Appointment with the Stork

A top priority of many working moms-to-be has become scheduling maternity leave and prearranging care for older siblings during the birth. With grandparents often living in other cities, plane tickets need to be purchased and maternity leaves maximized. Also, many women prefer to schedule a "daylight delivery" to ensure that their preferred OB-GYN will be present. It is common for hospitals in major cities to have induction rates over 35 percent.

But is this convenience for doctor and mom worth the risks? Many studies find that when labor is induced, the risk of a C-section doubles, especially in a first-time mother whose cervix may not dilate as quickly. Surveys have shown that many women are not informed of this risk before electing to induce. The highest rates of induction are during the month of December, of course. Should a doctor's vacation plans turn your little Capricorn baby into a Sagittarius?

Let's not dump all over the doctors here. We all realize that toward the end of pregnancy women are likely to say to themselves and to friends, and to scream from their bedroom windows, "I want this baby out of me!" You're sick of being so cumbersome, of being unable to reach the steering wheel because your belly is so damn big. So this is not just a modern phenomenon of trying to schedule the baby into our busy lives.

There are plenty of traditional, non-drug methods for trying to get labor started that have been passed down through the centuries. (In fact, women in the Listening to Mothers II survey found that 22 percent of women tried to self-induce.) Exercise is one. Sex is another (although honestly, are they kidding?). Women have also used castor oil or enemas to stimulate the digestive tract, release prostaglandins, which will induce labor, and empty the intestines so that the baby can shift into a better position.

Popular Natural Methods for Induction

There are many commonly used methods of natural induction, some supported by studies and other age-old methods that certain caregivers swear by. It goes without saying that you should never make an induction decision without first talking to your caregiver. Common methods include:

- Stimulating the nipples to release oxytocin and stimulate contractions.
- Sex. In her book *Ina May's Guide to Childbirth*, midwife Ina May Gaskin says that she and her partners have observed that women in their practice who were sexually active during pregnancy were more likely to go into labor at around forty weeks. Gaskin says that human semen is the most concentrated source of prostaglandins, which soften and thin the cervix in preparation for labor. Induction drugs such as Cervidil try to mimic prostaglandins. (Note that women who have had a history of miscarriage or premature birth should avoid sexual stimulation.)
- Castor oil or enemas. Both are used to stimulate the bowels and release prostaglandins. Castor oil is commonly mixed with fruit juice and called a "castor oil cocktail" by many midwives.
- Exercise. This can be as low impact as walking around your neighborhood. Movement will help move the baby down into a better position. Even if exercise doesn't induce your labor, a walk is probably good for you anyway.

Your caregiver probably has additional preferred methods. He or she may recommend acupuncture, acupressure, or certain herbs (black or blue cohosh are popular). Despite it sounding like an old wives' tale, some believe that going on a bumpy car ride can induce labor.

As we mentioned before, stimulating the nipples causes the body to release oxytocin and stimulate contractions. This is pretty powerful in some women, so those experienced with it recommend starting with only one nipple. Some midwives suggest stimulating the nipple with a

Bad Reasons to Induce

- You want this baby out of you. We know you are uncomfortable and huge, but it could be only a few more days until your baby is ready. The risks of inducing your baby are significant, namely the increased likelihood of getting a C-section.
- The ultrasound technician suddenly wants to move your due date closer, which means that you are already, according to them, overdue. These estimates are just that, estimates, especially at this late date. The estimates are accurate plus or minus three to four weeks in the last month of pregnancy.
- They tell you your baby is getting too big. They take an ultrasound of the baby and estimate the weight as bigger than eight and a half pounds. Keep in mind that these estimates aren't that accurate. They can be off by as much as two or three pounds.
- They tell you they need to get this baby out or your child might have shoulder dystocia, which is when the baby's shoulder gets stuck. But shoulder dystocia has more to do with the position of the baby than its weight. Babies are on the move all the time in labor. The baby might reposition or the problem can be handled via the Gaskin maneuver, in which the midwife positions you on all fours to allow the baby to move into a better position, or with other methods.
- Your doctor is leaving town or has scheduled a vacation and you want to deliver the baby while your doctor is on call. Remember, women who are induced have a higher incidence of C-sections.
- Your amniotic fluid is low. This drop in your fluid level can sometimes be countered by bed rest and drinking more water. Also it is just a rough estimate, not necessarily accurate.

breast pump for fifteen minutes, then taking a fifteen-minute break, and repeating this routine for an hour or two at a time.

Labor is a complicated process and it's not so easy to get it started in a way that won't potentially cause some harm to you or the baby. These days, the three most common methods of induction are the use of Pitocin, breaking the bag of waters, and stripping the membranes. Methods that fall in that middle zone between traditional and modern include breaking the bag of waters and stripping the membranes. A nurse, midwife, or doctor can use a device that looks like a crochet hook to puncture the membrane that contains the bag of waters. This starts the clock ticking for a C-section. Once the bag of waters breaks or is broken, most hospitals give you only twenty-four hours to be in active labor before inducing you, even if your baby is not in distress.

When the water breaks, there's an increased risk that infection will travel up into the uterus, particularly with all these people sticking their fingers in you to see how far you've dilated. Between 10 and 20 percent of women carry group B strep and breaking the bag of waters eliminates the protection from it. Your baby can pick up this bacteria if delivered vaginally or by C-section, and it is extremely harmful to a small number of babies.

Birth Goddess: Melissa Joan Hart

When actress Melissa Joan Hart was pregnant with her first child and preparing for the upcoming birth, she went into it expecting to fully embrace the experience. The oldest of eight kids, Melissa said, "My mom had all these babies, and I thought, 'She loved it, so I'm going to love it.' It wasn't that way, though. I just wasn't at home with being pregnant. It was strange and unfortunately it felt inconvenient to me. I didn't understand what was going on with my body." Melissa's baby was late, so she asked her doctor to induce.

"I was ready to just get my baby out and get my life going because I had been thinking about it for so long," she said. What followed was a difficult labor that lasted twenty-four hours. It took several attempts before the

(continued)

epidural was administered correctly. "They told me to start pushing, because I never had the urge. At one point, I had a forty-minute contraction, but luckily I had the epidural at that point—otherwise I would have been losing my mind." Melissa's doctor used a vacuum to assist. "There were three hours of pushing with my doctor saying, 'One more push and you're going for a C-section.' I kept saying no, but after all that time, I had no strength. Finally my mom said, 'I can see his ears!' and that made me go, 'Okay, his ears are here, his chin is here...' that finally got him out. The whole experience was really difficult and very medical. I did whatever the doctors and nurses wanted me to do." Melissa believes that her first son, Mason, just wasn't ready to be born at the time she was induced. "I think he would have stayed in there another two weeks. I was mentally ready to have the baby, and because it was my first, I wanted to be done with it and have that experience," she said.

When Melissa was pregnant with her second child, she wanted to do things differently. At a friend's recommendation, Melissa enrolled in Hypno-Birthing classes where she learned relaxation and visualization techniques. "What I took away from HypnoBirthing was the idea that you don't have to be a good patient. You don't have to do what the doctors and nurses tell you to do. They want to make it pain-free for you, and as easy as possible for them and for you. And they want to make you comfortable. But in Hypno-Birthing they teach you that birth is not a medical experience, and you have every right to bring the baby into the world however you want to, unless there's an emergency."

Melissa labored for nine hours at home, where she was able to doze off, take a shower, and walk around the backyard. When her contractions were slow, her husband would encourage her to get up and pace around the kitchen. "I got to be at home, and it was wonderful. I wasn't scared. When I felt a contraction coming on, I was able to relax," she said. In between contractions, her husband and mom would make jokes and they would all laugh together. "Finally someone made a joke and I started crying. I said, 'It's not funny!'" Based on this reaction, my mom could tell that I was in transition. She said, 'Okay, get in the car, it's time to go.' I had three contractions as I walked to the car."

Melissa had told her husband and mom that she wanted to try to give birth without drugs. She wasn't opposed to drugs, but she wanted to try it because she was expecting things to be easier the second time around. She felt that this time her body would know a little more about what to do. She was inspired by a friend who had avoided drugs by having her birth team urge her to wait just a little longer each time she asked for them—until the next contraction, for example. Eventually, her friend's baby was born, and she had done it without the drugs. "So I told my mom and husband that they might need to hold me off a little bit," Melissa said, "but if they thought it was going to be a long time, I didn't want to be a hero, so just give me the epidural."

Melissa checked into the hospital and labored on the toilet for some time. Then, she started asking for drugs. Each time, her birth team put her off. Things progressed quickly. To cope with the pain, Melissa made use of the techniques she had learned in HypnoBirthing. She and her husband had brought photos for her to use as focal points, but they didn't even have time to get them out. Her husband kept showing her a photo of their first son on his cell phone, which she used as her focal point. Melissa said, "I labored for a while more, leaning on the bed. My mom said, 'It's happening! It's happening!' I said, 'You're lying to me! That's what happened last time, and I was like that for six hours.' Then my husband whispered in my ear, 'You're nine centimeters. You're almost there,' and I was like 'Okay, okay, I can keep going.' They told me it was too late for an epidural."

Her doctor had Melissa lie down on the bed, and she told her that she needed to have a contraction while lying on her side with her legs closed. "It seems medieval and a little barbaric, but my doctor pushed my hip into the bed, so she was actually shoving my belly into the bed, which hurt like you would not believe. I remember hearing myself scream and thinking, 'I'm probably freaking out every pregnant woman on this floor,' but there was nothing I could do about it. Everyone flipped me over, and my doctor told me to push. What my doctor told me later was that the baby was turned a little; he wasn't quite sunny side up, but he was halfway, so with one push and one contraction, she got him turned the right way. And when he came out, he

(continued)

was ready. He was turned the right way. I felt everything. I felt where he had to go, and literally that was it."

Melissa was at the hospital for only an hour and a half before her son was born.

"Afterwards, my husband placed him right on my chest. I instantly started breast-feeding him. Physically, I felt great.

"The healing was so much faster and easier than with my first son. And while I don't think bringing a baby into this world is easy in any way, it is wonderful. I was fine and actually ready to do dishes very soon after my second birth. I was so excited to be at home enjoying time with my family. I felt so good so much sooner after my second birth thanks to a drug-free delivery and for that I thank my husband, mom, and team at the hospital."

The same cautions hold for stripping the membranes. This is a technique to start labor by which the doctor or midwife inserts her finger into your cervix and separates the amniotic sac from the inside edge of the cervix, which can stimulate the release of prostaglandins, another hormone that helps labor progress. Doing this can push group B strep up the vagina, which is why most midwives will not sweep the membranes of women who have tested positive for this bacteria.

Moving away from the traditional and mechanical ways of inducing labor, there are the pharmaceutical ones that doctors routinely recommend to advance a labor that they don't think is progressing quickly enough. Inductions are now so commonplace that we've developed this idea that doctors are god-like in their ability to wave a magic drug wand and start or stop labor at will. In reality, the drugs they use to prepare the cervix for birth and to stimulate contractions are crude tools when compared to the natural process of a self-started labor, but they are very effective. The problem is that once they get it going, it's really hard to pull back. As a result it's easy to hyperstimulate the uterus and give you contractions that slam you so hard that you're weeping. This can be painful and dangerous.

Another Option for Drug-Free Induction: Cervical Balloons

Okay, so your provider says that you need to be induced but you still want to avoid drugs. (See "Birth Goddess: Kellie Martin" on p. 189 as an example.) Well, in some cases induction of labor can also be accomplished through the less commonly used method of mechanical dilation with pressure. For many years some practitioners have used the inflatable balloon of a urinary catheter, called a Foley catheter, to exert pressure against the cervix. More recently, at least one biomedical company has introduced a product designed specifically for the purpose of cervical ripening. This device contains two separate inflatable chambers that place direct pressure against the cervical opening. Interestingly, this type of mechanical dilation of the cervix is associated with a decreased likelihood of uterine hyperstimulation and a decreased risk of cesarean delivery when compared with pharmacologic cervical ripening using Cervidil, Pitocin, or Cytotec. Given their benefits, why aren't these mechanical dilators used more often? Most likely, because human beings are creatures of habit. Doctors and midwives tend to use the techniques they know and the methods with which they are familiar. But ask your practitioner if he or she is familiar with balloon dilation of the cervix. If not, would he or she be willing to try it with you if you are a candidate for cervical ripening? The technique is easy, and you may help to effect change by suggesting the idea to your provider.

If the method of induction is Pitocin, they'll hook you up to an IV attached to two bags of fluid, one with hydrating fluid and the other with Pitocin, a synthetic version of oxytocin, which is the hormone naturally generated inside the pituitary gland to stimulate contractions. The staff can adjust the number of drops per minute you receive of the Pitocin so, if labor is moving too quickly, they can dial it back. The other bag of fluid can be used to flood you with liquid if your blood pressure starts to drop.

One change in your body that is essential for the smooth delivery of the baby is what they call the "ripening" of the cervix. The opening of the cervix needs to spread out and get shorter so that the baby has room to exit. The hormone that controls this is prostaglandin, one synthetic version of which is called Cervidil. The doctor can administer this on a strip that she stuffs up behind the cervix. There's a string attached to the strip so it can be withdrawn if things are moving along too quickly, but taking it out doesn't stop everything instantly because some of the medication remains behind.

If anyone suggests giving you Cytotec (misoprostol) to start your labor or ripen your cervix, inquire whether Cervidil is available instead. If the hospital only offers Cytotec, this may be preferable to using Pitocin on an unripe cervix, which carries its own risks.

Induction is part of the cascade of interventions. The augmented contractions usually require pain relief, which typically comes as an epidural. The epidural and the Pitocin battle it out for control of your womb, with the epidural slowing things down and the medical staff dialing up the Pitocin to get the contractions going again. If the staff can't get the drugs balanced right and this goes on for more than a couple of rounds without the baby emerging, you are getting closer to a C-section minute by minute. All of it increases the risks for the mother and the baby.

Good Reasons to Induce

- At forty-one or forty-one and a half weeks, the standard of care is to do an amniotic fluid index and a nonstress test (NST). If the fluid is genuinely low at this point, or the NST nonreassuring, some caregivers would consider this a valid reason for induction.
- If the baby is past forty-two weeks, trouble could be on the horizon. Like everything else, the placenta has a lifespan. Past forty-two weeks, it can start to break down, delivering less oxygen and nutrients to the baby. If the baby isn't moving around anymore, this is a good indication that the doctor should run further tests.

Additional reasons for induction can include:

- The baby is smaller than normal. This could mean that nutrients have been cut off to the baby.
- The bag of waters is broken but labor has not commenced. This can mean an increased risk of infection if not managed carefully. Most doctors will wait zero to six hours, while midwives will generally wait twenty-four hours before recommending induction. Of course, if the mom is strep B positive, the CDC recommends not waiting at all to induce.
- The baby is in distress, showing signs that oxygen has been cut off.
- If your blood pressure is spiking and there is protein in your urine, you may have preeclampsia. True preeclampsia can result in seizures. This, obviously, is a very serious condition and is a good indication for induction.

Another aspect of all of this that doesn't get much attention is how elective induction diminishes the baby's role in birth. The baby kicks off labor when she's ready to come, or so age-old wisdom shows. Some researchers say that when the baby's lungs are mature, she releases a hormonal signal that begins contractions. So if she doesn't release that signal and birth commences artificially, is she fully ready to greet the world? Augmented labor that produces blockbuster contractions sends the baby forcefully forward. This can create fetal distress, meaning spikes in the heart rate and meconium (the baby's first bowel movement) present in the amniotic fluid. These are other things that get the doctor recommending a C-section. When a contraction is spiking, there's very little blood flowing from the placenta to your baby. Contractions that come one right after the other, commonly caused by Pitocin, don't give you or your baby much of a chance to recover.

The quick progress of some induced labor can mean that not all parts of the process are ready for the baby to arrive. If the cervix is completely dilated and the baby has descended low enough but has trouble maneuvering the last little bit, the doctor may need to use a vacuum or forceps to pull the baby out. The doctor might use these methods if the descent of the baby has stalled and technological or other methods of progression have been ineffective. Pulling the baby out presents some risk to the head and pretty much guarantees you are going to have a vaginal tear or an episiotomy.

For all these reasons, think carefully before you agree to being induced or having your labor augmented by Pitocin. Don't let anyone rush you into this decision. Inductions are scheduled in advance, like some C-sections, which should allow you time to talk with your care-givers, your partner, and your doula and weigh the benefits and risks carefully before agreeing.

Questions to Ask before Being Induced

Unlike augmenting your labor with drugs to speed it up, induction is a planned event scheduled by you and your doctor. There is time to consider it carefully. Here are the questions you should ask:

Why are you suggesting induction?

What are the medical indications for it?

Is this drug approved by the FDA for use by pregnant women?

Are there special considerations related to my specific condition?

What is the scientific evidence that this drug or herb may make things worse?

What are the risks to me?

What are the risks to my baby?

What are the short-term consequences?

What are the long-term consequences?

How often do your patients need an epidural after taking this drug or herb?

How often do your patients need a C-section after taking this drug or herb?

How often do your patients require a vacuum extraction or forceps delivery after taking this drug or herb?

What are other possible solutions?

What are the risks or benefits of those other solutions?

What will happen if I don't do what you are suggesting?

(From Dr. Marsden Wagner's Creating Your Birth Plan*)*

10

Electronic Monitors
Reading between the Lines

In some ways birth in America is a survey course in accepting technology as a way to get a perfect baby. Technology tells you whether you are proceeding according to the average idea of how birth should unfold. The doctor doesn't spend as much time looking at you as he or she does looking at the numbers that describe your and your baby's condition.

It starts with the low-tech things like a blood pressure cuff and an electronic thermometer. As your pregnancy progresses, the more the technology increases with frequent ultrasounds, an amniocentesis, and blood tests. None of this can really assure you that you have a perfect baby, but as the readings and the measurements pile up, it sure begins to feel like you will. By the time women are on their way to the hospital for the birth, most fully comply with the idea that all aspects of the birth must be plotted on charts and follow graph lines to assure that things are progressing according to standards.

When the day of the birth arrives, it's a technology lollapalooza. Most women give birth on their backs attached to a tangle of wires and tubes. There are typically three bags hanging on the IV pole: one for the fluids (because you're not allowed to eat or drink), one for the epidural, and one for the Pitocin. There's a catheter in your urethra so you don't impede the progress of the baby by having a full bladder. The blood pressure cuff and the pulse oximeter record your vital signs, which are sent directly to the screens at the nurses' station. Perhaps the most important readout of all comes from the electronic fetal heart rate monitor (EFM).

Monitoring is standard in many hospitals. Usually when you enter the triage room, the belt for the fetal heart rate monitor is already spread out across the bed. The monitor has two sensors: the contraction sensor, or tocometer, which rests on your belly and gives you a little poke with every contraction, and the ultrasound device, which measures the baby's heart rate. Both of these are connected to a machine that thumps every time your baby's heart beats.

The idea behind this machine, invented by Dr. Edward Hon, an obstetrician who has retired from practice at the King/Drew Medical Center in Los Angeles, is that when the baby is deprived of oxygen, his heart rate will slow down. Being deprived of oxygen can cause serious damage to the baby. Dr. Hon believed that intermittent monitoring, done by simply listening to the mother's stomach with a Doppler, was not sufficient because it was not continuous and did not produce a printed record. He thought that for moms who had high-risk pregnancies, a second-by-second readout of the baby's heart rate would allow doctors to intervene quickly and thereby prevent many cases of cerebral palsy, mental retardation, and death.

If you're on Pitocin, there's a fifty-fifty chance that you'll be hooked up to an intrauterine pressure catheter because it produces a much better reading of the strength of your contractions. The doctor or midwife threads this catheter past the baby's head and up into your uterus between the baby and the uterine wall. When the uterus contracts, the pressure it places on the catheter is measured in millimeters of mercury, just like your blood pressure is. The strength of the contractions, which they plot on a graph, helps determine whether they need to increase the Pitocin. A woman's experience of her contractions does not count at all in this universe.

The fetal monitor often conflates the heart rate of the mom and the baby, so doctors looking for a more accurate readout choose the internal scalp electrode monitor, which is attached to the baby. Ricki had this for Milo's birth. The nurse straps a belt to your thigh and threads a sensor through your vagina, up your cervix, and into the uterus. When she hits your baby's scalp, she feels around to make sure that she's not attaching it to any of the soft spots in the skull. Then she screws the sensor to the baby's scalp. If you're curious what this might feel like to your baby, ask to try it on one of your fingers when they talk about monitoring at your birth class. We guarantee you'll give out a yelp. This monitor does produce much more accurate readings than the external monitor but, of course, is more invasive. This monitoring is only possible once your water has broken.

From the paper trail the doctor gets, which has a wavy line like an electrocardiogram, he or she makes a call about the condition of your baby and the quality of your contractions. If the baby's heart rate repeatedly drops in a way that the doctor considers abnormal, the doctor will start prepping the OR for a C-section.

Sounds fair if the baby is in distress, right?

Well, actually wrong.

In childbirth, the baby's heart rate can change dramatically from a simple shift in the mother's position. A dramatic change on the monitor can persuade the doctor that it's time for a C-section. "The EFM has been studied extensively and the results are clear. It does not prevent poor fetal outcomes," said Dr. Jacques Moritz, Abby's obstetrician, who practices in New York City. "What it does is lessen the need for one-on-one nursing and raise the rate of C-sections. If I monitored your heart for twenty-four hours beat for beat, trust me I would find something wrong. You add the lawyers who read these EFM strips with a fine-tooth comb in a courtroom and you have the American system in its full glory." In an article in *Boston* magazine in 2005, Dr. Laura Riley, director of Massachusetts General's labor and delivery department, called the EFM an embarrassment. "It's so ingrained now, and no one has the guts to pull back," Dr. Riley said.

As proof of this, the incidence of cerebral palsy has not decreased since the widespread use of the EFM began in the 1980s. Nor has all this monitoring improved the rates of mental retardation or seizures after birth. The number of C-sections for fetal distress has not gone down either, but the number attributed to prolonged labor has.

These readouts are frequently used to justify unnecessary C-sections when a glance at the printout of your contractions shows that your labor is not progressing according to insurance company guidelines or hospital protocols. Doctors do not want to open themselves to a lawsuit generated by allowing a labor to go forward that is even temporarily outside the range of fetal heart rate tolerances in the guidelines. All a lawyer would have to do to convince the jury of the doctor's malfeasance is wave the heart rate monitor strip under the jury's noses and point to the breaks in the hospital guidelines.

What this kind of monitoring also allows is supervision of labor by remote control. Each birth is as individual as each woman, and many healthy labors do not fall within corporate guidelines. The nurses are at the nurses' station, not in the room with you. They don't see any signs of distress in your face or your body posture. The only evidence they have of your condition comes from the readouts from the monitors that trace across the screen. The monitors measure the baby's heart rate but not the quality of those heartbeats. The best way for the medical profession to monitor childbirth is to have someone stay with the mother throughout labor and monitor how she is doing, checking the baby's heart rate every once in a while with a Doppler or fetascope. The graphs of fetal heart rate and contraction frequency produced on the screens at the nurses' station don't give a real picture of how the mom is progressing. Most hospitals unfortunately don't have enough staff to allow that.

There are some circumstances under which fetal monitoring is necessary—for example, if your labor is induced or if, during an initial examination on admission, the caregiver determines that there is a problem with the baby's heartbeat. An EFM is also standard when the baby is in the breech position, is premature, the mother suffers from high blood pressure or diabetes, the placenta is in an unusual position, or the labor is being augmented or induced with Pitocin. This monitoring is also standard for women who have epidurals or those who are trying for a vaginal birth after a C-section (VBAC).

If none of those conditions apply to you, the best way to make sure that your labor is on track is to have a caretaker who is skilled in listening to the subtle variations in the way a heart beats. With a stethoscope or a portable Doppler, an experienced nurse or midwife could detect the kind of variation that spells trouble. Hearing something this way is a lot different than viewing a readout from a remote monitor. This low-tech method requires frequent interaction with you but produces no long strip of readout that charts your baby's heart rate. Only by looking at you, and understanding the quality of your support system and the situation of the baby as she progresses, can a caregiver make an informed decision about whether a C-section is necessary.

But it's more than that, actually. The labor sped up or slowed down by drugs, the epidural, and the fetal heart rate monitor are each elements of the cascade of interventions that transforms you from the birth goddess to the birth vessel. The machines are in charge. Tethered to technology as you are by these things, your feelings about what is happening to you no longer guide the process. You might want to move around to help your labor progress, but no one is going to let you. You are immobilized and passive, waiting for the technology to deliver the baby to you.

When you choose a hospital or caregiver, it's best to ask if they allow intermittent fetal heart rate monitoring if you want to have more control over your labor and avoid a protocol-dictated C-section. If this kind of control is important to the way you envision the birth, you need to find a doctor, midwife, and a hospital that agree that this is important and can commit to helping you fulfill this desire.

11

Episiotomies, Vacuums, and Forceps
The (Un)Kindest Cut

There's a period in birth when some caregivers say you need to move quickly to get the baby out. To speed things along, the doctor may reach for a pair of surgical scissors and cut open the perineum, the tissue and muscle between your vagina and your anus. This operation is called an episiotomy.

An episiotomy is truly a woman's unkindest cut, as Henci Goer calls it in her book *The Thinking Woman's Guide to a Better Birth*. It can take months for the wound to heal and for you to be able to sit comfortably again. Doctors who do this intervention explain that they do it because it is the safest for the mother to ease her baby out into the world.

Except it isn't.

The reason some doctors and midwives prefer cutting a woman open to allowing her to tear naturally is that they say a tear is less safe than a cut and a smooth cut is easier for them to repair.

Except that's not true.

They also say that cutting the vagina protects it. The cut prevents the woman from experiencing urinary incontinence or vaginal or uterine prolapse and makes it more pleasurable to have sex later.

None of that is true either.

Maybe the doctors who still do episiotomies do so because they are surgeons and they like to cut things. Or because they are in the habit of doing it and don't like to break old habits. They sure aren't doing it because science has proven it's a good idea.

Even though there is no evidence that this cut in any way helps preserve the muscles of the vagina, 25 percent of women who answered the Listening to Mothers II survey reported that they'd had episiotomies. This is a big improvement over twenty years ago when the episiotomy rate in this country was 62 percent.

In the 1980s a group of studies tried to test out the basic assumptions that justify episiotomies. What they found revealed that the operation was essentially unnecessary. The baby is rarely in distress in the birth canal (which is what some doctors cite as the need for an episiotomy). This can happen to some babies, but most are just fine. Doctors have also said that babies sometimes damage their heads pounding on the perineum. Since the cut is made when the baby is nearly out of the vagina, this doesn't seem to make sense either. In fact, in a randomized trial of healthy, full-term babies, those born without episiotomies fared no worse than those whose mothers had one.

Midwife Tricks: Traditional Methods to Avoid an Episiotomy

- Allow the crowning of the baby's head to naturally stretch the vaginal opening. Some midwives will let the baby's head protract and retract for as long as an hour to gently stretch the perineum.
- Stay upright. When lying down to deliver your baby, gravity is not going to help you push.
- Push naturally, as your body guides you to do when the urge to push is undeniable. Coached pushing, when the staff charts your contractions on the monitor and cheers you on to push even if your body isn't telling you to do so, may force you to tear and can exhaust you. When you are tired, caregivers can suggest an episiotomy to help you get the baby out. You just might agree if you're exhausted.

> • Apply massage oil and warm compresses to the perineum—the space between your vagina and your anus where they cut you—to keep it soft and flexible during the second stage of labor.

Okay, so it's not the baby they're protecting. They're protecting the mom. When researchers examined that idea, they found it lacking too. Moms who had episiotomies in the previous generation, which was pretty much all of them, had plenty of incontinence and prolapses. And, as Henci Goer points out, how do you protect a muscle by cutting it? Cutting it doesn't make it stronger.

The last reason doctors typically give for doing episiotomies is that it is easier to repair a nice clean cut than it is to suture up a ragged tear. Even if that were true, would you tell your doctor that it's okay for him to cut you as much as he sees fit to get the baby out because it makes an easier repair? What if, when left untouched, you didn't tear at all? Or didn't tear nearly as much?

When women in the 1980s found out how barbaric and unnecessary episiotomies were, they started to object. Their consistent attention to this is the reason episiotomies have gone from the most commonly performed of all surgeries in 1987 to much further down the list.

Another reason doctors continue to justify episiotomies is their use of forceps and vacuum extraction delivery. They say that in order to get their instruments into the vagina and far enough inside to attach to the baby, they need more room to maneuver. Usually the motivation for doing this is that the hospital protocols have established a time limit on how long a woman is permitted to push and she has exceeded that limit. The staff may also have decided that she is not pushing effectively or that the baby is stuck and needs some help to exit. Yet, if the baby is not descending on its own, the skilled use of forceps or a vacuum-assisted delivery can spare you from a C-section. So the appropriate use of this equipment can also prevent more serious risks by avoiding surgery for mom and baby.

Forceps and vacuum extractors, when viewed outside the delivery

Craniosacral Therapy after a C-Section or Vacuum-Assisted Delivery

Babies who are pried from the womb or the birth canal can be traumatized by their birth. A vacuum-assisted delivery squeezes the delicate structures of the newborn skull, pulling fluid and tissue toward the top of the head. This, along with the twist and pull of the doctor's maneuvers, can cause a hemorrhage or a hematoma. Alternatively, the decompressive forces of the C-section may create similar physical effects on the newborn, like a scuba diver coming to the surface too quickly.

One way to counteract these effects is to take your newborn to see a craniosacral therapist. Craniosacral therapists use light-touch manual techniques to restore the central nervous system. A newborn can receive craniosacral therapy within minutes after delivery or up to several weeks later.

Dr. Steve Kravitz has performed craniosacral therapy on many newborns and finds that "correcting adverse mechanical tensions within the first few weeks after delivery, rather than later in life, may help avoid future problems caused during the child's maturation process including: digestive and elimination problems, musculoskeletal malalignments, respiratory disorders, sensory and motor defects, and learning disabilities." Ask your caregiver to recommend a craniosacral therapist in your area.

room, look as though they could be used in the kitchen or in a plumbing emergency. The forceps look like more elaborately designed barbecue tongs. Well, that's not exactly true. The mechanism is the same, but the shape of the tongs is unique. If you Google forceps to get images, some of them look like devices out of the Victorian medical cabinet of curiosities. They are oval-shaped with big spaces hollowed out in the center. Some have a brass mechanism with a screw handle that when turned regulates the distance between the tongs and holds that space steady.

The vacuum extractor looks like a tiny toilet plunger. The plunger is attached to the top of the baby's head when he's still up there inside you. A suction effect keeps the plunger attached to the baby's head, and the doctor pulls the baby forward by pulling on the handle of the device. (Usually doctors will make several attempts at this before deciding to do a C-section.) The baby is tightly encased in the soft, pliant, but strong muscles of the vagina and the uterus, getting a great body massage as he makes his way into the world. Your body isn't going to let just anyone interrupt that process before it's complete. Doctors need to pull with all their might. With forceps, though, it takes more skill, gripping tightly enough to grasp the head but not so much as to cause brain damage or damage to the facial nerves.

This is one reason forceps deliveries are no longer common in this country. The other reason is obstetrical programs no longer take the time to train new doctors in the delicate skill of forceps extraction when they can just perform a simple C-section instead. If the practitioner is highly skilled, forceps can be a lot more gentle than a vacuum extraction and can also be used to turn the baby into a more favorable position for a vaginal birth. Because so few doctors have the right touch with forceps (and the consequences are terrible if they don't), forceps delivery is no longer taught in most obstetrics programs. Dr. Moritz, Abby's obstetrician, says he wouldn't let anyone use forceps on his wife unless the doctor was in his sixties or seventies. He believes that this age group is the one with doctors who really know how to manipulate this tool. Dr. Stuart Fischbein agrees. "Forceps are almost dead in the water to the next generation of doctors, who lack any training in their use. Personally, I feel the loss of skilled doctors using forceps correctly will only increase the C-section rate."

As we've said, many women who get episiotomies aren't asked if they want one. In the Listening to Mothers II survey, 73 percent reported that no one asked them whether they wanted one. The best way to prevent yourself from having an episiotomy is to ask your caregiver what his or her episiotomy rate is. Anything north of 20 percent is cause for concern and perhaps even a reason to switch to a different caregiver. Episiotomies can be extremely painful and can be slow in healing. They also can increase the chances of incontinence, pain, and infection.

12

Cesarean Sections and VBAC

To C or Not to C

Ever since we started working together on the issues surrounding birth, it's been amazing to us how lightly people toss off the idea of having a cesarean section. They talk about it as if it's on the same level of complication as having an unsightly mole removed. In fact, C-sections are major abdominal surgery. This is a radical shift in the point of view the medical profession had about C-sections fifteen years ago, when doctors had to defend every C-section they performed as medically necessary. Now they must defend not doing one. Today, close to a third of all births end in a C-section.

When they take you into the OR for a C-section, most likely you're already hooked up to an epidural. All they have to do is increase the dose so that you are numb from the chest down. They shave your pubic hair, paint you with antiseptic, and put up a screen so you won't see the scalpel or breathe on your incision. If hospital policy allows, you can have your partner present. In some cases they allow another person there such as a midwife or a doula. In Abby's case Cara was there along with Paulo, holding her hand and describing moment by moment what was happening so that Abby could remain connected to the birth.

C-Section Myths

Doctors convince women to schedule C-sections by hauling out the following myths. We cite them here, along with explanations of why they are myths, so you can make up your own mind.

C-sections are safer than vaginal deliveries. The safest method of delivery for a healthy, low-risk mom and baby is a vaginal birth. All the studies support that.

A C-section prevents urinary incontinence and harm to your pelvic floor. A traumatic vaginal delivery can cause you harm, but most women don't have traumatic vaginal deliveries. Studies show that urinary incontinence rates were the same for vaginal births as for C-sections. Studies have shown that nuns, who obviously aren't having children, had the same incontinence rates as women who had delivered their babies vaginally.

C-sections are less traumatic for the baby. Babies born via C-section have a higher incidence of respiratory problems and are more likely to spend time in the neonatal intensive care unit.

C-sections are so much safer now; they're basically risk free. While it's true that C-sections are a lot safer than they were sixty years ago, the risk through anesthesia, damage to the bowel and bladder, risk to the baby, and postoperative pain, infections, and complications in subsequent pregnancies can't be ignored.

The C-section is necessary because the baby's cord is wrapped around the baby's neck. About a third of babies have the cord around the neck, sometimes wrapped two or three times. It's extremely rare that the cord is so tight or so short that a vaginal delivery will cause the baby harm.

(continued)

Once your water breaks—or is broken—you have to be in active labor within twenty-four hours. The hospital fears an infection can travel up the vagina and endanger the baby, who is no longer protected by the bag of waters. By limiting or eliminating vaginal exams, which can push bacteria into the uterus, you don't run much risk of infection. Caregivers who monitor the mom's temperature and make sure the baby is fine can safely establish that your labor is just taking its time without risk to you or your child.

To perform a C-section, the surgeon makes a four-inch horizontal incision right above your pubic bone through all the layers of the abdominal wall and into the cavity that contains your vital organs. This is not just one swift cut. He's got to make a bunch of smaller cuts through the interior muscles and tissues to get to the baby. Once the doctor gets through the skin and fat, he's got to cut through two leathery layers of fascia before he can see the uterus, which is underneath your bladder and bowel. He has to move those out of the way to slice open your uterus and get to the baby.

These Might Be Legitimate Reasons for a C-Section

- A prolapsed umbilical cord.
- Trouble with the placenta.
- Eclampsia (a very serious complication as evidenced by the mom having seizures).
- Inability for the baby's head to fit through the pelvis.
- Genuine fetal distress detected by a dramatic change in the baby's heart rate.
- Large tumor in the uterus that blocks the cervix as it opens.
- Outbreak of herpes at the outset of labor.
- Uterine rupture or previous uterine rupture.
- You're having twins that are not positioned head down.
- Your baby is in a transverse (or horizontal) position.

After he's made these cuts, he pushes down on your upper abdomen so he can separate the muscles and widen the opening into the uterus without cutting anymore. Through your dulled senses you will feel some tugging as he pulls out the baby. He clamps and cuts the umbilical cord and reaches in to peel the placenta off the uterine wall like peeling a pancake off a griddle.

The Honeymoon Vagina

One reason women give for electing to have a C-section instead of a vaginal birth is that they want to preserve the shape and resilience of their vaginas, the so-called Honeymoon Vagina.

The vagina was designed to stretch out and snap back. Men don't seem to have any problem with the idea that they have an organ that can expand dramatically (or not so dramatically) and then shrink back to its former puny size, but some women feel as though they have to apologize. Some even consider reconstructive surgery after a vaginal birth.

Dr. Jacques Moritz says that gynecologists can always tell just by looking whether or not a woman has delivered a baby vaginally. But men without such a practiced eye probably won't know the difference. The literature on this is inconclusive.

The major concern isn't so much the vagina, but what they call the pelvic floor, the muscles that support the pelvis, bladder, and intestines. These support the uterus in labor and also intensify orgasms if voluntarily squeezed during sex. These muscles stretch during pregnancy regardless of whether the baby exits your body via a C-section or through the vagina.

Do a Kegel right now. You know Kegels by now, right? Squeeze and release the muscles of your pelvic floor. Pay attention to the muscles that are engaged in that contraction of the vaginal muscles. In order to get that motion going, you've got to engage the abdominal muscles as well. If you have a C-section, the doctor must cut through those abdominal muscles, so no matter how you deliver the baby, the vagina will be affected. Fortunately, for most women, these muscles repair themselves within a year after birth.

(continued)

A study published in Canada in 2005 compared the sexual satisfaction of moms who had vaginal deliveries with those who had C-sections and found that 70 percent of the vaginal delivery moms were not happy with their sexual recovery compared to 55 percent of those who had C-sections. What wasn't highlighted as much is that episiotomies were a factor. Moms who delivered vaginally without getting cut had the highest sexual satisfaction overall.

For some women, the increase of blood supply to the vagina after a normal delivery enhances orgasm, and sex is actually better after a vaginal birth. The vagina isn't the only organ that controls sexual function either. The feeling of power and confidence that many women experience after childbirth also can improve a couple's sex life. And sex after a C-section can be painful, as some women who have a C-section suffer from abdominal pain and cramping for six to twelve months after birth.

In the end, it's difficult to say with any certainty what shape your sex life will be in after you have a baby. The good news is that with both kinds of pain and dysfunction, a good physiotherapist can guide you through exercises to restore your muscle tone and the integrity of your pelvic floor.

At this stage, there may be a bit of a delay before your baby makes a noise. The baby has been drugged by the anesthetic and has not received the benefit of the massage that comes while being delivered vaginally. Without the massage he would have received going through the birth canal that squeezes fluid out of his lungs, he has to work harder to take in his first breath. The nurses will rush him to be evaluated before you will be able to touch him. You'll remember that Abby was too out of it to touch Matteo when he was born, and anyway they had to rush him into the neonatal intensive care unit.

After the baby and the placenta are out, the doctor has to put you back together again. First he pulls your uterus outside your body and lays it on your stomach to get a good look at it while he stitches up the hole. This is the part when most women feel the most because for some unknown reason, the epidural doesn't handle this pain very well. The doctor stuffs the uterus back inside and positions it where it belongs, then tacks the bladder back into position, the fascia, and finally the skin. These days it's usually not stitches that put the skin back together. Doctors use staples or even tape.

If you consider the above description a bit of an over-share, we described it purposefully. A C-section is major surgery. Minor surgery is removing a mole. Major surgery is anything involving major internal organs, as clearly the C-section does, and should not be done without a lot of thought and consideration. Major surgery means the risk of major complications. When your doctor is cutting through so much muscle and tissue, and moving around major organs, the risk of infection and misalignment in healing are high, as are the risks to your baby. The risks increase the more children you have via C-section.

Lady, You Need a C-Section Because...

These are some of the legitimate and not-so-legitimate reasons a doctor might tell you that you should have a C-section. When you're in the hospital, drugged or not but certainly disoriented, doctors may try to persuade you that you are in need of a C-section when it's not necessarily true.

Your baby is too big. How does the doctor know this? Is it from an ultrasound? Those readings can be wildly inaccurate—off by as much as two or three pounds. And while it is true that babies have gotten bigger over the last few decades, that alone does not determine whether your baby can safely be born vaginally.

Your pelvis is too small. A substantial percentage of women are told that their pelvis isn't big enough for a baby to pass through. The clinical term for this is cephalo-pelvic disproportion. How does the doctor establish this? Midwife Ina May Gaskin believes that standard U.S. obstetric thought has been based upon some misapprehensions about the capacities of women's bodies in labor and birth. The pelvis changes dimensions in response to the movement of the baby during birth. If the baby does not descend despite strong, regular contractions, your pelvis may be too small for the size of the

(continued)

baby's head. However, Ina May observed that she and her colleagues have encountered fewer than eight such cases in approximately twenty-five hundred births, suggesting that there are likely to be other factors involved in the reasons so many U.S. women are having cesareans.

You wear only a size six shoe. Some old-fashioned doctors make a guess about the size of your pelvis based on the size shoe you wear. Does that sound right to you?

Your baby is not happy. What a crock! That baby doesn't know anything about happiness or unhappiness yet. What does the doctor mean by that? Ask for signs that your baby is actually in distress.

We need to get this baby out. Again, ask for actual signs of distress, not just medical staff impatience. Keep in mind that studies show there is a spike in C-sections around 4 p.m. and at 10 p.m., which is when doctors want to go home for dinner or to bed.

You don't want to hurt your baby, do you? This is called "Playing the Dead Baby Card." No mother would want to run even the smallest risk of hurting her baby. But is the situation of the labor in fact harmful? If you are exhausted and frustrated, it may be hard for you to ask the questions necessary to establish this. This is where a well-informed partner or a level-headed doula can be very helpful.

You have an active infection in the vagina that can harm the baby. If the doctor has detected an active herpes lesion in the birth canal, this is an indication for a C-section.

Your baby has stopped growing or is not moving as much. This is a sign that the placenta may be degrading or the cord is tangled. Doctors usually try an induction first.

Your baby is breech. The standard of practice now is to deliver breech babies via C-section, although some midwives and doctors still practice the skill of breech delivery.

Celebrities like Victoria Beckham and Christina Aguilera endorsed the convenience of elective C-sections when they announced that they had their babies that way. Posh Spice, married to David Beckham, scheduled the deliveries of her three children to work with her husband's soccer schedule. As Christina Aguilera, who scheduled her C-section when she was thirty-seven weeks along, told *People*, her stresses weren't about her husband's schedule, but more about deciding what would be the best birthday for her child. As she said, "I didn't want any surprises. Honestly, I didn't want any [vaginal] tearing. I had heard horror stories of women going in and having to have an emergency C-section [anyway]. The hardest part was deciding on his birthday. I wanted to leave it up to fate, but at the same time I was ready to be done early!"

Breast-Feeding and C-Sections

In recent years there has been a resurgence of interest in breast-feeding. In fact, the American Academy of Pediatrics has issued policy statements recommending that the optimal nutrition for most infants is human breast milk, and most pediatricians would agree that exclusive breast-feeding for the first six months of life is highly desirable to ensure proper growth and nutrition.

A study published in the professional journal *Pediatrics* in 2003 examined some of the factors that might be associated with suboptimal breast-feeding. One of these factors was found to be delivery by cesarean section. If there is a lack of immediate bonding between mother and infant, this could lead to a delay in initiation of breast-feeding. This also might occur due to the increased use of analgesics in the postpartum period.

Almost all the research on this subject shows that anything other than an unmedicated birth impacts the rate of breast-feeding, the success of establishing breast-feeding, and the duration. However, these results may contain an innate bias as the women that tend to go for natural birth are usually more motivated to breast-feed. Mothers delivering by C-section should be aware that they may need extra support from family and lactation consultants to ensure successful breast-feeding.

It's also true that some companies offer a longer maternity leave for new moms who have had C-sections (since it is surgery), which could also play a role in women making this choice. That extra time off, at home with the new baby, can be tempting.

In April 2008 a *Time* magazine story entitled "Choosy Mothers Choose Caesareans" estimated that between 4 and 18 percent of the dramatic increase in C-sections in the last twelve years has been women electing to have them. That's a pretty big point spread, making it essentially a guess (and directly contradicting the Listening to Mothers II survey, which found one woman out of 1,600 surveyed had scheduled a purely elective C-section without any medical indication). The article also guessed that for modern women, "childbirth was losing some of its magic." Birth, they quoted an expert as saying, had become more about getting the baby out safely than experiencing the miracle of life.

Hang on a second. That assumes that having a C-section is safer than "experiencing the miracle of life." It's not.

C-Section Risks

For some women with high-risk situations, like Abby, C-sections are medically necessary and can even save the life of the mother or the baby in a true emergency. We cite the risks here to help you avoid being talked into an unnecessary C-section. These are the downsides that low-risk mothers should consider when a C-section is optional or elective. In high-risk situations or emergencies, obviously the benefits outweigh the risks.

- Although the risk of dying is small in either form of birth, a woman is five to seven times more likely to die from a C-section than from a vaginal delivery. Twice as many women have to return to the hospital after a C-section than those who delivery vaginally. They suffer infections, blood clots, hemorrhages, blood poisoning, and trouble with scars not healing well. The antibiotics they take for these infections can interfere with breast-feeding.

- Babies born to low-risk mothers via C-section are three times more likely to die; close to two per thousand babies born via C-section die compared to only one out of every two thousand babies delivered vaginally.
- Two out of every hundred babies born via C-section are nicked when the doctor is slicing into the womb.
- Babies born via an elective C-section are four times more likely to have persistent respiratory problems and jaundice, and are three times more likely to be confined to a neonatal intensive care unit. This separation from the mom at the crucial first moments after birth can interfere with their forming a close and immediate bond.
- Having a C-section could affect your ability to get affordable health insurance even years later. A July 2008 *New York Times* article reported on several women who were denied coverage and/or charged higher rates for individual coverage because they'd had a C-section. Having a C-section greatly increases the chances that your next birth will be a C-section, which is more expensive for your insurance company. The *Times* reported that some insurance companies, such as Blue Cross/ Blue Shield of Florida, increase your premiums by 25 percent for five years as a hedge against the expense of your next C-section.

The World Health Organization says there is no evidence that any time the C-section rate in a country goes above 10 to 15 percent that it is saving lives. WHO examined the infant and maternal mortality rates around the world. They found that poor countries with C-section rates below 10 percent had high infant and mother mortality, but in countries with a C-section rate above 15 percent, the rates were even higher. If you believe the WHO determination about the proper number of C-sections, that would mean that U.S. women have more than double the optimal rate for C-sections with its nationwide rate of 31 percent. This may be why the United States has some of the worst mom and baby outcomes in the developed world.

Even if you believe the 4 to 18 percent estimate from the *Time* article, it would not explain why C-sections have doubled in the last twelve years. It's clear that doctors order the vast majority of C-sections. Doctors now order C-sections for breech babies and twins, the kinds of babies they routinely delivered vaginally way back in the 1970s. Back then the national C-section rate was 5 percent. In many obstetric programs, C-sections have become so routine, students aren't taught how to deliver these kinds of babies vaginally. The biggest factor in the increase in C-section is not that, however. The rise in primary cesareans (for first-time moms) accounts for slightly more than half (about 53%) of this increase and the other half (47%) is caused by the catastrophic drop in the number of vaginal births after an original C-section, commonly called VBAC.

Having a vaginal birth for your second child after the first one was delivered via C-section used to be standard. Doctors encouraged it. Now you have to search hard to find a hospital that will allow you to have a vaginal delivery after a C-section.

Your Best C-Section

If you have to have a C-section, how do you make it as mother-friendly and baby-welcoming as possible?

"You want to eat steak three times a day," joked Cynthia Flynn, a Washington midwife who is the president of the American Association of Birth Centers. What she means is that you should have as high a blood iron count as possible. There's a lot of blood loss in a C-section. Perhaps she's recommending the Atkins diet, because she also advises not to gain too much weight as belly fat makes it harder for the doctor to cut and creates space for infection.

Cynthia also advises, if it's possible, to wait for labor to start before you go in for the section. At that point the baby is closer to being ready to come out and will get at least the hormonal benefits of the early stages of labor.

For one planned C-section Cynthia assisted at, she negotiated in advance with the hospital to ensure that her client's mother and husband could be in the room during the operation and that she could bring the baby in to visit the mom in the recovery area so she could nurse. Normally the baby would be taken to a nursery and the mom would not be able to nurse until she was out of recovery.

Heather Baker set out to create the best C-section for herself and her babies when she discovered at thirty-four weeks that one of her twins was breech, which guaranteed she would be having a C-section. She ended up doing a lot of what Cynthia recommended.

Although Heather loved her obstetrician, her feeling was that lines of communication might get crossed at the hospital. The doctor gets focused on the operation and she wanted her husband to be able to relax and focus on her. She hired a C-section doula.

"The doula would be our advocate in whatever way that meant," Heather said. "She could get me something to drink or get someone who needed to come into the room. I knew I wanted to nurse the twins right away and she could help with that. She could do whatever I needed at that moment."

The doula met Heather and her husband at the hospital. Whenever they had a question, she got the answer. She was also a labor and delivery nurse at that hospital, so she had a good relationship with the hospital staff and was allowed into the delivery room where she talked Heather through the whole operation.

Once Heather was out of recovery, her doula made sure that the twins were nearby for the initial breast-feeding. She also helped arrange for Heather to get a private room.

Dr. Jacques Moritz has performed C-sections where he tried to make the operating room as calm and serene as possible, considering what was going on. Instead of the bright lights, jocular music, and shouted orders that a lot of surgeons favor, he kept the general lighting low and asked the staff to speak in muted voices to make the baby's entry into the world a bit more gentle.

This all started in 1996. Prior to that, every organization from the federal government to the obstetrician's society ACOG encouraged VBAC. A study of VBAC women published in the *New England Journal of Medicine* that year showed that women attempting a VBAC had twice the risk of complications. Three times as many women's uteruses ruptured with a VBAC than with a primary cesarean, and when the woman was induced that figure shot up to six times as many.

But wait, how could that be true when Dr. Bruce Flamm, an advocate of a more reasonable, evidence-based position on VBAC, couldn't find any data to support that as he reported his research in his book *Birth after Cesarean*. He reviewed thirty-five years' of studies on the subject that collectively logged the results of eleven thousand women. In all of those studies, not one woman died from a uterine rupture. Turns out that the doctors disagree on what exactly a uterine rupture is.

Uterine rupture is a frightening idea, something right out of *Alien*. That your stomach could burst open and expel your baby into the world is something that every woman would go to great lengths to avoid. That's what is known as a complete uterine rupture. Some say that a partial uterine rupture, where only a bit of the tissue separates, doesn't do any harm to the mother or the baby (although others disagree and there is a controversy that surrounds this). Dr. Flamm found that in some studies, they lumped the two types together to come up with their alarming conclusions.

Certainly a real uterine rupture is a terrifying thing. When the scar from the previous C-section separates inside during labor and contractions move the baby up against that weak point, thereby forcing it further apart, if the baby is not out within an average of fourteen minutes, it can cause brain damage or even death. Dr. Stuart Fischbein, a Los Angeles-area obstetrician, says that if a clinician is watching carefully, he or she often will be able to see the signs of an impending uterine rupture half an hour or more before it happens and get the woman into surgery in time to save her baby and her uterus.

After the *NEJM* study was published, ACOG issued a series of recommendations over the next four years that narrowly defined the circumstances of a woman who should be allowed to have a VBAC. She should be a healthy woman whose average-weight baby is coming basically on her due date and whose previous C-section was not because her labor had failed to progress. She should have had no more than one previous C-section and should have her baby at a hospital that has an operating room prepped and an anesthesiologist ready twenty-four hours a day. This meant that VBACs were no longer possible for women who fell outside that exacting criteria and who didn't live near large, fully staffed hospitals.

U.S. Cesarean Rates

1970	5.5%	
1975	10.4%	
1980	16.5%	
1985	22.7%	
1990	22.7%	
1994	21.2%	
1995	20.8%	ACOG recommends VBAC for most women
1996	20.7%	*New England Journal of Medicine* article says VBAC dangerous
1997	20.8%	
1998	21.2%	ACOG reverses its position on VBAC
1999	22.0%	
2000	22.9%	
2001	24.4%	
2002	26.1%	
2003	27.6%	
2004	29.1%	
2005	30.2%	
2006	31.1%	

Suddenly the percentage of VBACs dropped dramatically. After the legal ramifications of the study sank in, women found it almost impossible to get a doctor who would attend them for one. VBACs were close to 30 percent of births in the years before the *NEJM* study was published. Now they comprise 7 percent with a corresponding spike in the number of C-sections.

Birth Goddess: Andie Smith

When people talk about the way birth transforms a mother, they're often talking about natural childbirth. If that's what they're referring to, they miss the way a C-section can change a modest, people-pleasing woman into an outspoken advocate for herself and for other women.

This is what happened to New York state mom Andie Smith after she was persuaded she needed an unnecessary C-section.

She had been frightened of labor so when the doctor suggested an induction she agreed, thinking it would give her more control over the experience. The doctor justified the operation by telling her that her baby was too big for her small frame. The baby would be at least eight pounds and Andie is a very petite woman who had only gained twenty-three pounds during her pregnancy. Every woman in her family delivered five-pound babies.

Andie was induced with Pitocin and Cervidil, but because her baby wasn't ready to be born, the contractions caused fetal distress that resulted in a C-section. Afterwards, the staff wouldn't let her hold her baby and mismanaged her pain medication. "I really didn't get to hold her and put her by my heart. They had to sew me back up. I didn't get to see her for a few hours, maybe even more when I was in the recovery room. I was the only one screaming after giving birth," she said. "My family felt bad for me."

Later Andie was relieved that it was over and that her baby, who turned out to weigh five pounds thirteen ounces, was all right. As the months wore on she got more and more upset by the thick red scar at her bikini line, which she called her "angry scar." She was even angrier when she found out how hard it would be for her to have a vaginal birth after a C-section.

When she was pregnant with her second child, she went from doctor to doctor in her county trying to find one who would let her labor naturally. All of them tried to scare her off with warnings about the hazards of VBAC. Her determination to do the second birth the way she wanted it changed her inside. She continued her search until she found a supportive group of doulas and midwives and a retired doctor who all cheered her on.

The VBAC labor was much different. Andie was not afraid this time. "Being out of control felt like being in control," she said. "It wasn't as painful as most people make it out to be. I just went to this place inside myself and just zoned out and I felt my body. I had complete trust in my body and the process. During my labor I felt supported and taken care of. I did not feel like a liability or a legal risk. Instead, I felt embraced as a woman in labor who trusted her body. Everyone in the room was rooting for me."

The baby was born with no complications and Andie has a new respect for her body. As she said, "During my search, I learned that our society worships fear and control and does not trust women to do what has been a natural process since the beginning of time. If you ask women who have had C-sections why they did so, most will say that something was wrong with them. But today's woman is the same as yesterday's woman. All that has changed is that our society has invested in the medicalization of birth, and lost its confidence in women along the way."

Multiple C-sections introduce new difficulties. Each time they cut into your uterus to get your baby, the scar tissue that built up from the last C-section complicates things. That scar tissue makes it tougher to cut in, increasing the chances of C-section injuries and complications. The accumulation of scar tissue on the uterus can also make it more difficult for you to get pregnant the next time. It also increases the chances that any subsequent pregnancy will have difficulty with getting the placenta to fully attach or having it grow over the cervix or into the cervix, something called placenta accreta.

With all these complications and risks and murky science supporting the increase in the number of C-sections, why are doctors insisting on them so frequently?

The old doctor's tale that is passed around from doctor to doctor is that the only C-section you are ever sued for is the one you didn't do. Just as with the VBAC, the hospital protocols have defined a very narrow standard for what is considered a normal birth. Twenty-four hours past the breaking of the waters means an induction, which means a much higher chance of your having a C-section. Generally, a woman who is not dilating a centimeter every two hours is a C-section. These strict ideas of how birth should progress determine whether a woman who is having a conventional hospital birth will be able to deliver her baby vaginally.

The baby may not be in a moment of distress, but the doctor doesn't want to get sued. Even a misjudgment on the part of the doctor that results in a lawsuit can boost his malpractice rates dramatically, so many doctors can express impatience with a mom-to-be's fixation on vaginal birth. It's interesting, the paradox created by the medical model of childbirth. The gadgets and gizmos, the readouts, and test results seem to guarantee that this scientifically precise monitoring will produce a perfect baby. When the baby comes out less than perfect, the mom is more likely to want to blame the doctor.

We hope you'll consider all of this if your caregiver recommends a C-section. And, if a VBAC is what you're after, we encourage you to make your wishes known, advocate for yourself, and work with your caregiver to make it happen.

The Slow Cesarean

Speed seems to be the most important concern in the C-section, with the whole operation very impersonal.

In response to this, Dr. Nick Fisk, an obstetrician in the United Kingdom, has pioneered something he calls the skin-to-skin cesarean. As detailed in an article published in the British newspaper the *Guardian* in December 2005, Dr. Fisk decried the fact that even with planned C-sections, the parents never got a chance to participate in the arrival of their baby. The skin-to-skin C-section is different in the following ways:

- The drape that typically obscures a mom's view of her body is withdrawn as the baby emerges so she can see her baby being born.
- At first, only the baby's head is removed from the uterus, allowing the baby to receive a few minutes of the benefit of a body massage as the uterus contracts.

- Instead of quickly clamping and cutting the cord, the doctor leaves it intact and allows the baby to slowly acclimatize to the surroundings with support from the placenta's blood and oxygen.
- As the baby seems to become more alert, the doctor hands the baby to the mom, who places her little newborn on her chest for skin-to-skin contact. This way bonding can begin. The baby awakens to the world hearing Mom's voice and smelling Mom's smell instead of being on a resuscitation table.

Mothers whose C-sections follow this procedure seem to get a better start on family life, midwife Jenny Smith told the *Guardian*. "Breast-feeding is easier to establish, and you can see how much calmer the baby is."

TAKE BACK
YOUR BIRTH

Well, we've arrived at labor, the destination of this amazing journey you've been on. There are few events of life when you are so intensely involved for such a short time and get such a spectacular result. Don't be scared. It's going to be fine. You've prepared perfectly. You've read up on all the things that might try to derail your plan. You've chosen a great support team and a place to give birth where you feel comfortable. Soon the baby, that longed-for baby, will be in your arms. So let's demystify and celebrate this labor. How do they always describe luck? As a time when preparation meets opportunity. Well, lucky you. You're going to have your baby.

As you know by now, our culture makes labor seem scary and mysterious. Part of the problem is the weird mix of modern medical language, Greek words, and evocative terms used by the medical establishment that make it sound surreal. There's the "bloody show," a term that, heard out of context, conjures up images from horror films or *Sweeney Todd*.

And there's the "breaking of the waters." Have you ever seen water break?

The term "trial of labor" is imprecise too. Surely you and those around you will be tested during this trial. Your relationships with those you love, your endurance, your pain threshold, all of it comes into play during childbirth. Yet it progresses fastest and with the least complications when you yield to the natural course of labor and essentially do nothing. As perinatal educator Karen Strange says, normal birth is designed to work when there is no one else there, just as it did before doctors and hospitals came into being.

Traditional remedies that have been handed down from woman to woman across the centuries stand right alongside the drugs and electronic hardware of modern medicine. The gadgets and readouts are another way to mask the fact that for the overwhelming majority of women, labor goes smoothly and the old techniques work remarkably well.

The World Health Organization says that 70 to 80 percent of labors commence with a mother who is considered to be low risk, and only when there is a valid reason should caregivers intervene. Even if you have a high-risk pregnancy, you can have an uncomplicated labor. The goal of all caregivers should be the stated objective of the World Health Organization: to have a healthy mother and baby with the fewest possible interventions.

World Health Organization Recommendations for the Best Birth

- The well-being of the new mother must be ensured through free access of a chosen member of her family during birth and throughout the postnatal period. In addition, the health team must provide emotional support.
- Women must participate in decisions about their birth experiences.

- The healthy newborn must remain with the mother whenever possible.
- Immediate breast-feeding should be encouraged even before the mother leaves the delivery room. Unrestricted mother-infant contact after delivery and unrestricted breast-feeding reduce breast-feeding failure.
- There is no justification for a hospital to have a caesarean section rate of higher than 10–15%. Vaginal deliveries after a caesarean section should be encouraged.
- Electronic fetal monitoring should not be routine.
- There is no indication for shaving pubic hair before delivery.
- There is no indication for routine enemas before delivery.
- The dorsal lithotomy position during labour and delivery is not recommended. Women must decide which position to adopt for delivery.
- Induction of labour should be reserved for specific medical indications.
- The routine administration of analgesic or anaesthetic drugs should be avoided.
- Artificial early rupture of membranes, as a routine process, is not justifiable.
- Enhanced social and psychological support from caregivers reduces negative outcomes. Leaving women unattended during labour should be abandoned.
- Separating healthy mothers and babies routinely should be abandoned.
- Repeating caesarean section routinely after previous caesarean section should be abandoned.
- Restricted maternal position during labour and delivery should be abandoned. Upright versus recumbent position during first and second stage reduces negative outcome.
- Performing episiotomy routinely should be abandoned.
- Inducing labour routinely at less than 42 weeks gestation should be abandoned.
- Prescribing sedatives or tranquilizers routinely should be abandoned.

Labor can stall, however, calling for interventions to get it moving, and judgments related to what is progress and what is really a stall are the reason for many C-sections. Between 20 and 30 percent of C-sections arise when labor stalls, according to the standards of hospital protocols, and a doctor gets impatient and wants to "wrap it up" or predicts disaster. As you will see from this story of labor we are about to detail, when you prepare yourself emotionally and physically and choose the people around you for birth carefully, you give yourself the best chance of avoiding interventions and common labor procedures that can interfere with your baby's progress.

We've been describing a kind of childbirth throughout this book that, we hope, is centered on you and your baby and exactly the situation in which both of you would feel the most supported and the most comfortable. This idea of labor and birth insists that you think things through for yourself and decide what you believe to be best. In addition to that, we want you to go out and get exactly what you want, like a good consumer. Once you've examined all your choices, talked them over with your partner, and surrounded yourself with an environment and a team that you believe can handle whatever comes up, you have the right and, in fact, the responsibility to completely relax and simply birth your baby.

The Birth Goddess: Having a More Natural Birth with Each Baby

Sarah Ulrich's amazing story is one that will inspire you if you're feeling discouraged about your past experiences and how they will play into your upcoming birth, because it shows that you really can create your own version of your best birth.

When she was pregnant with her first daughter, the Lancaster, Pennsylvania, resident's planned home birth turned into what she called "a nightmare emergency C-section." After laboring for hours at home, and pushing to no avail, her midwife saw what she called "unsettling bleeding" and arranged for an ambulance to take her to the hospital. When the doctor there examined her, he said the baby's head had not descended properly and that Sarah needed an emergency C-section. Other interventions were not presented as options, but Sarah was so tired and out of it that she agreed.

She was depressed about the C-section for months afterwards. "When you get in your head that you want a natural childbirth, an emergency C-section feels like the ultimate failure," she said. "I eventually came to terms with it, but I struggled for a while, and was angry with myself that I had such a mind–body disconnect when I was in labor."

Sarah knew that if she had another baby, she wanted to have it naturally. When she was pregnant again, she called several midwives and learned that none of them would take a first VBAC at home. When she went to one local obstetrics practice that had midwives on staff, they had her sign forms up front with a list of points that they would not be responsible for during labor. "The message was that they would try a VBAC with me, but they would probably fail," she said. It left her feeling more scared than anything. Eventually she found a practice with midwives on staff where the understanding was that a VBAC was a possibility, and there was no reason why Sarah shouldn't try.

She was still a little worried that her body wouldn't be able to do it. "I didn't want to be that woman who ran to the hospital every time I tried to have a home birth," she said. So she decided to birth in the hospital with a midwife. She and her partner visited the hospital several times before Sarah was due and got themselves used to the idea of having a hospital birth.

When she had gone into labor and arrived at the hospital with her partner, the midwife met them there. Without Pitocin or an epidural, Sarah labored on her hands and knees, with her midwife at her side. Sarah was able to have a successful VBAC with no interventions.

"With my first birth, I woke up afterwards feeling groggy and traumatized. My second was so much better. I was up on my feet, and I got to hold my baby right away," she said.

"When I was pregnant the third time, I started out assuming that no caregiver would want to take me at home. I took Bradley classes again with my partner (I had also taken them during my first pregnancy). My teacher

(continued)

had had several babies at home. Her experiences got me in the mood for a home birth again, because it reminded me of what natural childbirth is all about, and what my body was capable of. When I was twenty-eight weeks pregnant, we decided on a home birth. We just went for it."

Sarah found a midwife with her own practice who did home births, and who was able to do a VBAC at home—just as long as it was a second VBAC.

"Having my prenatal visits at home and getting to know my midwife ahead of time made a real difference," Sarah said.

When she went into labor and her contractions were just a few minutes apart, it was midnight and Sarah called her midwife. Her baby was born almost three hours later, with Sarah's eight-year-old daughter alongside them (she had asked to be woken up for the birth).

"The midwife didn't cut the cord right away, and she let me hold the baby while she checked us out and stitched up my tear," she said. Her baby started breast-feeding right away. Then, the midwife tucked them all into bed and went home.

"I was so much happier with this birth," Sarah said. "I was comfortable being in my own home with the midwife, and it seemed more natural to me that my older girls could be in the room with us when she came for follow-up visits. They'll be adult women some day, and it's important for them to see that childbirth isn't something to be afraid of."

Looking back at her three very different experiences, Sarah says that the most important lesson was learning to trust that her body could do it. "It's one thing to read about natural childbirth. It's another thing to really meditate on it, and understand that you can and will do it. Every birth is different, and you have to realize that your birth will happen in the way that it's supposed to happen. You need to go with the flow, and try not to have too many expectations about the birth. If I hadn't been so rigid about my first birth, I think I would have felt more at peace about it afterwards. You have to pay attention to your body. No matter who else is there, in the end it's really just you. You're in it by yourself. It's just you and your body trying to do this amazing thing, birthing that baby."

You can be as passive or as active as you want. You can have pain relief or do it naturally. Whatever it is you decide, your body will, in the overwhelming majority of circumstances, produce a healthy baby and an exhausted but ecstatic mom. We're going to begin this section by focusing on the story of one mom, Michelle Macis, who prepared for labor in exactly the way we recommend. You'll find that because she was so well-prepared and had thought things out so carefully, her daughter, Isadora, had the best birth possible. In fact, it was miraculous not only for them but also in the way it affected her entire family.

13

Loving Your Labor

Michelle Macis's pregnancy wasn't planned, but she took control of it soon thereafter. Michelle has always believed that she should trust her body, and she didn't think it should be any different in labor. She expected that her womb would perform the task it was designed to do without her trying to interfere with the process. Also, she's distrustful of hospitals, so she and her partner, Nick Homan, chose to go to Community Childbearing Institute, the only birth center in San Francisco, for her initial prenatal care and for the birth.

Her attitude toward health care, and pretty much everything else, has made Michelle a bit out of step with her immediate family. She grew up in the suburbs of Los Angeles with a father who was an LAPD officer, a family with pretty typical American aspirations. Her sister, Jennifer Morrison, following her dad's strict sense of order, became a navy nurse stationed in Virginia. Michelle moved to San Francisco, a city her father had never visited because he despises its unconventional attitudes and politics.

"The age difference is so big that there's never been much rivalry, but there's always been a wall between us," said Michelle of her sister, who is seven years older.

Additionally, Michelle had been distant with her dad, who got divorced from her mom when Michelle was two years old. Michelle's best friend, Heather, whom she's known since they met in kindergarten, now remembers their teenage spring break visits to Michelle's dad, who had retired to Arizona, with humor. "We were the school poets, writing angst-ridden poetry. My hair was dyed blue and I spent the trip trying to convince him his politics were wrong. You can imagine how all of this went over," she said.

In her prenatal classes at Community Childbearing Institute, Michelle worked with the childbirth educators to understand the risks and advantages of a fully natural birth in the birth center. Prominent in her mind was her sister's emergency C-section, which their mother had witnessed.

Jennifer had wanted a natural delivery, too, but she had a lot of meconium in her water when it broke and her epidural only worked on the right side of her pelvis, causing her excruciating pain. Her emotions were high, as was her fear. Labor stalled so she ended up with a C-section. Michelle did not want to end up in the same situation as Jennifer, who had, at one point, eight navy doctors staring back at her from her crotch consulting about what would be the best course for this birth. This was an idea that really frightened Michelle.

She was also in turmoil about which members of her family, if any, she wanted to have with her in labor. In many ways, Michelle was going to use the birth to show her skeptical family that her approach to things had been right all along. Not that she actually wanted to show them the birth. After much consideration of her emotional state and the various forces in motion in her family, Michelle decided that she only wanted Nick and Heather and Nick's mom attending her at the birth. She scheduled her family's visit so that they would arrive after the baby was born.

The problem with this plan was that the baby was eleven days late and, when Michelle went into labor, her whole family was still in San Francisco.

This brings up the problem of relying on due dates. There is wisdom and mysticism in the mechanism that brings a baby into the world, a natural sequence of events where one movement releases a hormone that stimulates a muscle that brings the baby gradually and elegantly another small step closer to entering the world. The baby and the mother work together to create the proper circumstances for birth. It's not a process that responds to anyone's timetable, however.

In the last six weeks of pregnancy the baby, who has been flipping and twirling in the pond of amniotic fluid, gets too big to perform these acrobatics. Influenced by the natural forces of gravity and motion, she positions herself head down, the largest part of her nestled in the cradle of the pelvis. All during your pregnancy, the ligaments and cartilage that hold your pelvis tight have been receiving doses of the hormone relaxin to encourage them to create more elasticity in your lower back, pelvis, and pubic bone. This situation remains fluid and the baby keeps shifting even as she is settling into the head-down position.

Penny Simkin's Five *P*s of Stalled Labor

In Penny Simkin and Ruth Ancheta's *Labor Progress Handbook*, a technical manual for midwives and doulas, they draw on their vast experience and training to simplify ways to get labor unstuck, including numerous illustrations of positions women can take to get that baby to move into the right position. This is their clever summation of the different factors in the body and mind of the pregnant mom and her baby that can bring labor to a halt. Obstetricians learn the first three in medical school, but Penny and Ruth added two that we think are just as important.

The powers (the uterine contractions).

The passage (the size, shape, and joint mobility of the pelvis and the stretch and resilience of the vaginal canal).

The passenger (the size and shape of the baby's head, presentation, and position).

The pain (and the woman's ability to cope with it).

The psyche (the anxiety, emotional state of the woman).

The optimum situation for labor is a woman who has increasingly power-ful, regular contractions that move her average-sized baby out of the uterus and into the world. Ideally she is able to cope with the pain of this process and has dealt with any emotional issues that labor or delivery might present prior to the day of the birth.

She's quite a little acrobat, your baby. As she wiggles further down, sometimes pushing off against whatever firm structures are handy, she gets her little arms in the tuck position. She's hunkering down, getting ready for the big moment when she's going to draw her first breath on her own.

As the baby moves down, the uterus starts to adjust the baby's posi-tion, so that these movements will propel her gradually down the birth canal. As we mentioned, studies show that when the baby's lungs are developed, they secrete a hormone that kicks off the contractions.

While the baby is moving into position, the cervix is starting to do what the caregivers call ripen. The cervix is the neck, or opening, to the uterus and is a powerful ring of muscle. It has to be powerful in order to keep the opening closed during the time when the baby is growing in the womb. When the baby is mature enough to be born, the cervix begins to thin out and soften, in preparation for labor. Midwife Ina May Gaskin describes the cervix as similar to the cord that holds a drawstring purse closed. Labor is actually the process of the opening of the cervical ring of muscle until the baby's head is able to move through it, much as a head moves through the neck of a turtleneck sweater.

If this is your first baby and you go in for one of those frequent pre-natal exams close to the due date, your caregiver will be assessing the state of ripening as a way to predict when you're going to have the baby. If they tell you that you're two centimeters dilated and labor is going to begin within twenty-four hours, don't get too excited about that. The

Birthing from Within: Birth as Self-Expression

A central idea of this philosophy of childbirth is that "active, creative self-expression is critical to childbirth preparation." This method asks parents to write journals, do sculptures, and engage with other art forms to explore their fears and feelings about birth and the baby to come. Check this out if you're compelled to explore your feelings about your upcoming birth through a creative lens.

The *Birthing from Within* book is full of reproductions of parents' birth art. The parents are not exactly Picasso, which is nice to see because then you won't be so self-conscious if your drawing looks like it was made by your baby, instead of by a fully formed, allegedly motor-coordinated adult.

Birthing from Within addresses the physiological aspects of birth but the focus here is on the expression and getting these ideas out into the world. The emotions portrayed in these pieces can be surprising, and seeing them expressed can make it easier for you to explore them with a bit of distance.

condition of your cervix is not a great predictor of the onset of labor. While the ripening of the cervix and the intensifying of contractions are both essential, they're not linked. The ripening of the cervix in the late part of pregnancy doesn't cause contractions to begin, but during labor the stronger contractions help the cervix to open. In this, your body is going to do what it's going to do and getting fixated on someone else's timetable can lead to disappointment and anxiety.

In the first phase of labor, the contractions are light, just a tightening, and not particularly painful or regular. It's a nice time when you can putter around the house, maybe cook a little, and clean if you feel like preparing the house for the arrival of the baby. Michelle's sister, Jennifer, remembered the burst of energy she had just before she went into labor, when she sensed that the baby would be born within twenty-four hours.

This energy and restlessness is good for the baby. The more you move around, the more the baby edges into position. The contractions gradually intensify as the uterus starts its work. This is why when Michelle called Judi Tinkelenberg, a certified nurse-midwife and the owner of Community Childbearing Institute, late on Saturday night to tell her that she was in labor, Judi wanted specifics about the contractions. Even Dr. Emmanuel Friedman, whose Friedman Curve is used by doctors and hospitals to pinpoint whether labor has stalled or not, has said that there's no way to distinguish real labor from false labor except in hindsight.

Judi said it sounded too early in labor for Michelle to come to the birth center, and recommended she call her doula, Rachel Engel, to be by her side. By nine the next morning, labor was progressing nicely and Judi told Michelle she'd meet her at the birth center.

Birth Classes: Why Don't Parents Go?

In the last few decades childbirth classes have been as much a part of preparing for birth as picking out the crib. The classes give couples a general survey of anatomy, including what's happening as the baby grows, and how to manage pain during labor. Classes taught at a hospital also tend to review the various interventions used in the one-size-fits-all hospital birth. Yet lately fewer and fewer couples are attending these classes. Depending on the hospital, attendance at classes has fallen off by as much as 50 percent in recent years.

This may be because couples are exploring different birthing philosophies, such as Lamaze, Bradley, Birthing from Within, and HypnoBirthing, that typically aren't covered in hospital classes.

Some women who plan to get an epidural are advised that they don't need to learn the coping techniques taught at these classes. This seems dumb, honestly. Clearly there is a lot more to birth than just blocking out the pain. As birth educator Erica Lyon, who runs Realbirth in New York City, observes, there is no other area in our lives where we would so easily give over the decision making. "Many people spend more time researching the stroller than they do trying to understand the physicality and the emotional-loadedness of getting a baby out of their bodies," she said. And a good birth class might actually change your mind about some of the things you didn't consider.

(continued)

No matter which of the various classes you decide to attend, the impor-tant thing is to remember again that this is your birth. You should ask as many questions as occur to you and never think that what bothers you might be considered a dumb question. It's likely that other people in the class have the same question.

If you're not engaged, these classes are like all those boring classes you took in high school where you didn't retain a single fact as soon as the final test was complete. When Listening to Mothers II survey asked moms about birth classes, most of them were extremely happy they had attended. But when the survey quizzed them about basic aspects of childbirth, most moms gave the wrong answers!

Lyon, who wrote *The Big Book of Birth*, a coping manual for pregnant moms, recommends staying away from the hospital birth classes. The teach-ers there are frequently under pressure from the hospital administration to edit the instruction they give couples to reflect the kind of birth choices that the administrators want them to make, such as getting the epidural.

A sure sign that the class is being controlled from the boardroom is when the teacher is not allowed to give couples her phone number or e-mail address if they have follow-up questions. This means that the hospital is afraid private communications might stray from the approved curriculum. Erica was "called on the carpet" when she mentioned at a hospital birth class she taught that some women suffer light itching after an epidural. While the anesthesiologists were fine with her mentioning this side effect, the hospital was not.

Look for classes that limit enrollment to no more than ten couples and take up fifteen total hours of class time. Erica believes that's the minimum time necessary to educate couples in all their choices as well as coach them in some effective coping techniques. "Massage is a tool; privacy is a tool; vocalizing, breath work is a tool; visualization is a tool. This is why I don't believe there is a method. It's like telling people there is a method for sex," she said.

Equally important to what couples learn is the friends they make and, through those relationships, how they begin to get a better idea of their best birth. "A woman might believe that her doctor doesn't spend any time with her and the visits are really rushed and that is just how it is," Erica said. "When she is in the class with people who are under the care of other doctors and midwives she finds out that in other practices the practitioner spends an hour with them. It's a grassroots way of learning how to advocate for yourself."

Let's just have a small detour here to talk about how amazing the uterus is. As midwife Ina May Gaskin points out, if men had such an organ, they would be bragging about it to everyone they knew. No other organ of the body can do what the uterus does during the course of pregnancy and birth. At the beginning of pregnancy, the uterus is about the size of a pear, and by the end of a single pregnancy, it is more like the size of a large watermelon. The strongest muscle of the body, the cervix then starts contracting at intervals as it opens to allow the expulsion of the baby, which then moves down the birth canal. After the birth of the baby and delivery of the placenta, the uterus contracts down to its original size.

In fact the uterus is the only organ in the body that can generate new cells as it expands; those cells are reabsorbed into the tissue as the uterus shrinks down after the baby is born. During the strong contractions of labor, the uterus produces seven hundred pounds of pressure per square inch. At that time it's the strongest muscle in the body. This is why it is especially cruel to read how on ultrasound reports technicians characterize a normal uterus as "unremarkable." For some legal reason they can't call it normal, but if they were being honest, they'd call it incredible.

Midwife Tricks: Stay Hydrated with Laborade

Midwives generally believe women need to eat and drink to keep their energy up during labor. Some midwives give women diluted hydration drinks like Recharge to keep their electrolytes replenished. Trish Fox, a New York City doula, makes what she calls Labor Aid, a concoction of one-third cup

(continued)

agave nectar (or to taste), juice of half a lemon, a quarter teaspoon of salt and baking soda, and enough water added to this to make a quart of fluid. Trish thinks this is a great alternative to sports drinks that include high fructose corn syrup and can cause heartburn and nausea.

By the end of pregnancy, the uterus is huge! The top of it is bumping up against your stomach and pushing past the lower rib cage. At the end of the pregnancy, these muscles are stretched thin across the top of the amniotic sac, but they are still powerful and maintain an incredible capacity to contract to push the baby toward the world. Even after being so stretched out to the size of a watermelon for so many months, within minutes of birth, the uterus will have returned to the size of a grapefruit and six weeks later back to where it was before you got pregnant. As the uterus contracts, the baby cooperates by doing her part.

Dr. Michel Odent: First Do Nothing

French obstetrician Michel Odent thinks exactly the opposite of the way American doctors do about women giving birth. He wants us to discover how easy and uncomplicated birth can be if, instead of rushing and testing and preparing, we just let it happen.

He is fond of recalling the traditional midwife: a woman who would simply sit in the corner knitting unless called for. She is there to guide and reassure if she's needed, but her presence should be as low-key as possible.

As he details in *Birth Reborn*, in the 1950s, Dr. Odent was assigned to be the head of surgery in a small hospital in the French countryside, where he was also needed to perform the C-sections, which were just becoming popular as a "rescue operation." As he studied the midwives' techniques, he began to think that the safest births would take place in a quiet, dark room much like a room at home, where a woman could forget she was in the hospital and concentrate on her labor.

The innovations he developed at that hospital, including the homey birthing suite, gradually have been adopted by hospitals all over the world. He's the one who pioneered the use of a small children's pool to help women with the pain of contractions, the precursor of birthing tubs. Dr. Odent is a big fan of home birth too.

He's also done groundbreaking research into the cocktail of hormones that work in combination to make labor progress or stall. He firmly believes that how babies are treated in the womb and how they are born affects their health and well-being for the rest of their lives.

When everyone entered the birth center around 10:30 in the morning, there was a lot of tension in the air. Lois, Michelle and Jennifer's mom, and Joe, their dad, as well as Jennifer, were seated in the lounge area while the moans of Michelle's labor punctuated the air. Joe looked tense. "I'm kind of old school," he said with a worried look on his tanned face. "I'm the kind of guy who likes this sort of thing to be in a hospital." Jennifer looked like she was going to jump out of her skin. She wanted to be in the birthing suite with her sister, but Michelle had told her she only wanted Heather and Nick and Nick's mom there. Of the three of the family in the waiting room, only Lois seemed content to be that far away from her daughter. "Just the sound of this is killing me," she said. "I hate hearing my baby in pain."

In the birthing suite, although Michelle was the focus of everyone's attention, she was oblivious. She was in the birthing tub, a blue tiled whirlpool built about two feet off the floor, with steps leading up to it and a ledge around the base so attendants could have a place to stand. No lights were on in the room, whose pale blue walls were illuminated by the sunlight filtering through the frosted glass. An inflatable pillow wrapped in a towel supported Michelle's head. Her eyes were closed and she seemed as if she'd arrived at Labor Land. As the contractions came, she breathed deeply into them and let out long, low moans of surrender. Later she would remember how vivid and nearly psychedelic her dreams were when she was in the tub.

He He He He Hooooo: The Way a Bit of Breath Transformed Birth

The scary films about childbirth often feature women breathing hard with puffed-out cheeks, eyes wild with anxiety. These are parodies of what was a groundbreaking method of helping women cope with the pain of childbirth, the Lamaze method, which revolutionized birth sixty years ago.

The 1950s was the dark ages for natural childbirth. Women were separated from their husbands and led into maternity wards where they were knocked out and later presented with their babies. Late in the 1950s an American woman named Marjorie Karmel gave birth using a focused breathing technique developed by French obstetrician Fernand Lamaze to help her handle the pain. She wrote a book about it called *Thank You, Dr. Lamaze*, and the idea of giving birth naturally started to spread. Dr. Lamaze also encouraged fathers to be in the room during labor to help coach mothers in their breathing.

By the 1980s the Lamaze method was a standard part of many hospital birth classes. In the two decades since then, the organization has moved away from the focus on a simple breath technique and toward advocating a whole philosophy of pregnancy, birth, and parenting.

This is not your mother's Lamaze class.

Lamaze still teaches three separate breathing techniques for different phases of labor, but it also advocates a philosophy of birth that follows seven simple principles:

- Birth is normal, natural, and healthy.
- The experience of birth profoundly affects women and their families.
- Women's inner wisdom guides them through birth.
- Women's confidence and ability to give birth are either enhanced or diminished by the care provider and place of birth.
- Women have the right to give birth free from routine medical interventions.
- Birth can safely take place in homes, birth centers, and hospitals.

- Childbirth education empowers women to make informed choices in health care, to assume responsibility for their health, and to trust their inner wisdom.

Women who study the Lamaze principles will get tips on trusting their bodies throughout pregnancy, strategies for how to hold to their idea of natural childbirth during birth, and support for the formation of a stronger family.

After each contraction, Judi reminded the doulas to have Michelle take a sip of water so she could stay hydrated.

It is hard not to compare this scene with all that we know about what the typical hospital birth is like, as described in the beginning of the book. Had Michelle been laboring in a hospital, she would not be allowed to eat or drink and, most likely, she'd be hooked up to at least the fetal heart rate monitor, the pulse oximeter, and the blood pressure cuff. Attached to those, the tableau would be very different. All the focus in this birthing suite was on Michelle because there were no dials or readouts to consult. Judi said she felt no need to give Michelle a vaginal exam, as they would be able to hear and see when she had moved into the pushing phase of labor. "This is not something you can rush. It has to come on its own time," Judi told Michelle. "You've made huge progress since you got here."

Between contractions, it almost seemed as though Michelle were asleep, deep within herself, waiting for the body to make the next move. At the end of each contraction, the chorus of encouragement erupted. "Relax and open," said the midwife-in-training, Shannon Stalock, who attended the birth. "Can you feel the baby is pushing forward on its own? Relax and open."

The Bradley Method

The Bradley Method has been around for about the last fifty years and is now recommended by many physicians and used by couples around the world. It is a type of natural childbirth that promotes a drug-free birth via relaxation techniques, deep abdominal breathing, and a relationship between the woman and her partner in which he plays a very active role in the birth. The Bradley Method encourages what is called "love talk" between the woman and her partner during childbirth, building intimacy and morale, and even laughing in the birthing room—all with the aim of making labor easier for the woman, reducing pain, and promoting bonding between the couple and the baby.

Bradley classes are taught nationwide (check the Resources in the back of this book or look online for classes in your area). Classes are typically small and focus on birthing and relaxation techniques. They also coach you in helpful positions and ways your partner can make you more comfortable while helping you stay optimistic and focused before birth and as labor progresses.

As the due date approaches, the Bradley Method recommends daily drills of envisioning and rehearsing for labor, and practicing relaxation techniques so that when the big day comes, you both are confident that you know precisely what to do.

Judi recommended that Michelle shift from side to side to relieve the pressure on her butt. Every few contractions, Shannon placed the Doppler at Michelle's pubic area to take a reading of the baby's heart rate. Half an hour into this phase of contractions, Michelle stood up and started to do a squat as she rode through another contraction with the doulas holding her arms to keep her from slipping. When the next contraction came, she was on her knees. The doulas had placed a doubled towel at the edge of the tub so she could rest her elbows. "Sink into it," Judi said, as Michelle let out a rising moan.

Suddenly Jennifer appeared in the birthing suite, tentatively at first.

She hovered on the periphery, watching with a sharp eye to see what the birth attendants were up to. This brave act of coming where she was not invited created an unaccustomed awkwardness in her. She's a strong, sunny personality who wants to be useful, but she didn't know quite what she was supposed to do. Then Lois, Jennifer and Michelle's mom, entered carrying with her a similar combination of concern and discomfort.

The doulas aided Michelle to open her pelvis by supporting her in a modified lunge: one knee on the seat inside the tub and the other knee extended to the side and held up by Rachel so Michelle's pelvis was completely open, and then switching sides for the next contraction.

With each contraction, the women in the room murmured encouragement in their own ways.

"Good, good," Lois said. "You're doing swell."

"C'mon, go for it," cheered Jennifer.

Things seemed to be moving very quickly and then they slowed. The contractions were farther apart and less intense. The mood of the room shifted downward to a watchful quiet. Judi suggested nipple stimulation to get things moving again and, as everyone but Nick started to leave the room, Michelle asked her sister to stay. On her way out, Lois pointed to the oxygen tank and said, "Oh good. I'm glad they have that. I'm gonna need it."

In the lounge, when Joe was informed that the group left so that his daughter's nipples could be stimulated, his eyebrows shot up as his eyes widened. "Oh!" he said. "You know, when my daughters were born, I was in a room with a lot of other fathers and we were all pretty grateful that we couldn't hear a thing." Some people were in the kitchen fixing themselves a snack, but the most nervous of all appeared to be Lois. "I'm a wreck!" she announced.

A few minutes later, the sound of a long moan that rose to a huge peak notified her family that Michelle had another contraction. All the women went back to the birthing room to see Michelle exiting the tub with Nick on one side and Jennifer on the other. The magnificence of that beautiful full belly was hard to deny. Aided by her supporters, she took grand and delicate steps down from the edge of the tub.

Midwife Tricks: The Cocktail Stop

When a woman has gone into labor too early, midwives will recommend they have a glass of wine or a shot of vodka. Alcohol can slow labor down. Be aware that it makes many women nauseous.

By noon Judi believed that the only thing that was preventing the baby from making her entrance was Michelle's full bladder. "It's like the baby is pounding her head on a trampoline," Judi said. She asked Michelle, who was having trouble urinating, if she would like Judi to insert a catheter to drain her bladder. "The baby will probably be out pretty quickly after you do that." Michelle agreed.

About an hour later, Michelle was being guided how to sit on the birthing stool, a small, open seat on legs that supports the laboring mom's weight but leaves plenty of room for her to open up for birth. Judi asked Michelle if she wanted Nick to catch the baby or if she would prefer that he support her. Michelle wanted his support, so he took his place on a regular stool behind her, holding her elbows with a pillow positioned on his chest to cushion her.

The energy in the room was electric as the contractions started to come more quickly. Nowhere was this more apparent than with Jennifer, whose manner changed dramatically. She had been cheering her sister on with sports phrases like, "You're almost at the finish line!" and later, "Atta girl! Come on!" When the baby's head started to be visible, Jennifer spoke much differently to her sister. "You are so beautiful," she said with a waver of emotion in her voice. "I love you so much. You're awesome."

As Michelle sat on the stool, you could see the way the contractions rippled across the surface of her belly. The baby had dropped quickly with all the space freed up by the empty bladder. Minute by minute, the top of her abdomen shrunk back to a prepregnancy shape as the lower part of her belly expanded just a bit more.

"You feel the baby down there?" Shannon asked.

"No," said Michelle, who would collapse into Nick's arms, her head slack on his shoulder as she rested between contractions.

"You don't feel it? We can see the top of the baby's head!"

"I don't know what I feel," Michelle said.

The contractions were stronger and closer together, less than two minutes apart. The effort/rest cycle of Michelle's labor was breathtaking. The sounds she made were fierce, coming from a place of power, desire, and exasperation. She worked each contraction so hard that all across the top of her clavicle was flushed a beautiful rose color. Periodically Shannon would check the baby's heart rate with the Doppler and call it out, a number between 100 and 110.

Birth Goddess: Kellie Martin

Actress Kellie Martin says that having a baby was the biggest thing to ever happen in her life. "Giving birth naturally was a very big goal for me," she said. "I don't know why I initially wanted it. I think it was partly because my mom and my mother-in-law both gave birth naturally. I was like, 'If my mom could do it, I can totally do it.' I did everything I possibly could to stick to that goal." Kellie enrolled in HypnoBirthing classes, prepared a birth plan, and hired a doula. Kellie was drawn to the breathing techniques that HypnoBirthing offered (she is a yoga person), as well as the meditation. She says she took what she needed from it (some of the visualizations didn't work for her, for instance), and in the end it just resonated with her. Kellie had considered giving birth at home, but she said she wasn't quite brave enough. So she planned for a hospital birth, and packed her own music, pillow, and nightgown (although she didn't end up wearing it).

Kellie was almost two weeks late. "I was enormous," she said. Although she agreed to an induction, Kellie was adamant that she didn't want Pitocin. At the hospital, the nurse gave her the option of Pitocin or induction with a cervical balloon (without Pitocin). She opted for the balloon, which was inserted into her cervix, where it mechanically opened her two to three centimeters. She also had a cervix ripener (a gel swab that softens the cervix). The balloon

(continued)

and cervix ripener started her active labor. Afterwards, Kellie's water still wouldn't break. "My body was just not willing to have this child," she said.

Her doula arrived at the hospital and connected Kellie with the labor and delivery nurse, who was known to be very supportive of natural childbirth. They broke her water. "Once they broke my water, my contractions got humungous in the span of a minute," Kellie said. "It was like *boom*. I was on the birthing ball, and I looked up at my husband, and said, 'I need an epidural right this second. I can't do this.' My husband and the nurse just changed the subject. My contractions just kept coming and coming, and I forgot about it. I realized that I just had to manage them. I wanted to move around, and I also spent a lot of time sitting on the toilet. And then I knew when it was time. I didn't think I wanted to give birth in bed, but I went to the bed, and my nurse and husband just followed me. I got in a fetal position, and I knew it was time to push. It was kind of magical. I was so with my higher power. I was praying. My sister passed away ten years ago, and I was talking to her. I don't think anyone knew I was talking to her, but I had my guardian angel, I had God, and I was having my baby. I feel like I was able to go through all of those sensations because I was blessed. I was able to give birth naturally."

Kellie pushed for twenty minutes, but the cord was wrapped around the baby's neck. They put oxygen on Kellie's face. "My husband is the calmest man I've ever met," she said. "I know when he's getting a little nervous because he's incredibly calm. He looked at me, and he got really close, and he said, 'She needs to come out right now.' I took the oxygen off and I said, 'I can't push any harder than I'm already pushing.' He said, 'Yes, you can.' I put the oxygen back on and I was like, 'All right.' And I got her out because she needed to come out.

"When Maggie was born, she was amazingly alert. She was just there, and she wasn't groggy," Kellie said. "I felt amazing afterwards, and relieved, and also kind of stunned at how enormous she was. My recovery was amazing, too. We don't know what our bodies are capable of until we give birth. Then you look at it and you go, 'Holy shit! I didn't know that could happen.' Women have had natural childbirth for centuries. This is what women did when they didn't have drugs. You can do it. We're built for it. That's what I learned—that I'm built for this."

Soon Michelle's water broke. She screamed in pain with every contraction as the crown of the baby's head was visible.

"Let it sit there," Judi coaxed. "Let it stretch you. Let it stretch your tissues."

"You're a strong pusher, Michelle," Jennifer said. "You are unbelievably strong."

"And it's okay to cry," added Judi.

One of the things that Michelle was the most concerned about was that she not tear. Judi was trying to deliver the baby's head gradually, allowing the head to slowly stretch the vaginal tissues out, if Michelle could stand to wait for it. If she did it slowly, the chances of a tear would be greatly diminished.

Midwife Tricks: The Rebozo

A traditional midwife often carries with her a big Mexican shawl called a rebozo that can help if a woman is in back labor (meaning that the baby faces toward your pubic bone with skull pressing against your spine. Agony!). She places it under the mother's pelvis and uses it to elevate her butt to move the baby out of the pelvis and into a more favorable position in the pelvis. This can also work to jumpstart contractions that are inefficient.

"You are so strong," said Jennifer. "Keep breathing. I am so proud of you."

"Everyone in this room can see your baby's head," said Judi. "Can you see?"

Michelle threw her hands up in frustration and confusion and shook her head no because she could not see her baby's head, when she was suddenly rocked by another contraction.

"You're stretching your tissues beautifully!" said Judi. "A little push. A little push." Judi reached in around the baby's neck. "No cord. No umbilical cord around the neck."

In a surreal moment, the baby, whose head was completely free, started to move her head around. Then, with one big push at 1:18 p.m., Isadora came out into the world and up into her mother's arms with a grand gurgling scream of pure new life. Everyone in the room was crying. Even Joe, who had been standing with a stricken face in the doorway around the corner from the action, was overcome. He couldn't enter the room because Michelle hadn't yet delivered the placenta and was still seated on the birthing stool, and in his traditional, formal way, it didn't seem right to him to see his daughter like that.

"She's perfect," Lois said. "She's absolutely perfect."

"How much does the baby weigh?" Joe wanted to know.

Judi craned her head around the corner. "We're going to wait on that for a few hours," she said. "No baby ever died from not being weighed."

Days later when most of the family was scattered back to their respective homes, the glow of this birth still had a transformative effect. Joe, who lives in Arizona, had to leave first. His plane reservation was for that same night. Days after the birth, he seemed to have gained a new understanding of his daughter. "You know, I've learned I've got to accept my daughter for who she is," he said. "She's going to live in San Francisco and have her baby in a place that looks like a storefront because that's what she wants to do and it's going to be all right with me. For me, I'm a conservative who wants everything done by the book and I could not be more pleased. It was a real eye-opener."

But the person who seemed the most affected by the experience outside of Michelle, Nick, and Isadora was Jennifer. "I feel like I have my little sister back," Jennifer said. "I was so grateful to be there and happy that she trusted me and she relied on me. I texted her today and I said, 'You just amaze me.' That's a big thing for me and her."

For Michelle, bathed in the baby-bonding hormones as she was in the week after the birth, the whole experience was perfect. She was fully prepared and more supported than she could have ever anticipated.

HypnoBirthing

HypnoBirthing® is a powerful yet simple method that promotes relaxation during pregnancy and childbirth by releasing conscious and subconscious fears. The idea is that when we are afraid, our muscles constrict causing pain, which in turn brings on more fear. HypnoBirthing aims to break the Fear-Tension-Pain Syndrome.

HypnoBirthing is a complete childbirth education course that covers pregnancy, childbirth, and parenting. You learn specific breathing techniques and self-hypnosis to take you into a relaxed state and create your body's own natural anesthesia. The course includes training in visualization, preventing vaginal tearing, creating birth plans, and communicating with your doctor, midwife, and hospital staff.

Alisha Tamburri, a clinical hypnotherapist and doula in California (www .HypnoBirthingCA.com), says that "hundreds of couples in my classes have had the births they imagined; blissful, empowering, and a calm baby." She now has many obstetricians enrolling in her classes for their own births, after they've seen how well their patients were able to manage labor using the HypnoBirthing techniques.

Some midwives and doulas feel that moms who study HypnoBirthing may derive benefits from taking the course but are often disappointed when they start to experience pain during their labors. These midwives and doulas warn clients not to harbor a false expectation that their births will be painless and then feel discouraged when they are not.

14

Bonding with Baby

Renee Ostellino had three other children, the third born at home, so she was confident going into the birth of her fourth child with two midwives attending her at home. When her baby's head emerged, she heard one of her midwives say, "I've got cord. I've got short, tight cord." Renee wanted to be coached as to what to do to help her baby. "I was ready to do whatever it took to get my baby through this. I was asked to be still while the more experienced midwife coached my other midwife on clamping and cutting. They told me not to push but it went against everything I was thinking. I wasn't prepared to do nothing. No pushing, no movement. When I was finally told to push, I drew a deep breath and propelled my baby into the waiting hands of my midwives," she remembers.

There was an eerie silence in the room while the midwives flicked their fingers lightly on the soles of her daughter's feet and told her to breathe. Kathy, the more experienced midwife, said, "Talk to her, Renee."

Renee called to her, not knowing if she was her son or daughter. "Wake up baby! Come on, wake up. Time to meet your family." That's when Renee heard her cry. The midwives waved oxygen under her nose.

Weeks later, Renee brought her daughter Abigail to the pediatrician. When Renee placed her on the examination table, Abigail turned to follow her while she stepped aside to let the doctor examine her. He commented on how Abigail's eyes followed Renee across the room and how rare that was at her stage of development. He also commented on how bonded she was to her. "To this day, eight years later, we still hold a unique bond," Renee said. "Had she been born in a hospital, she would have been whisked away to be treated by professionals who would have underestimated the bond between mother and baby."

Postpartum Holistic Comfort: Arnica

Arnica is a homeopathic remedy for bruises and muscle soreness that has been used for five hundred years. The arnica plant grows about two feet tall and produces bright yellow flowers. These flowers produce a substance that can be consumed in a pill or distributed in a cream that can be rubbed on the parts of you that have been stretched to their maximum during childbirth.

Arnica is also used to stop bleeding, and some claim it's mentally soothing too. Arnica is very safe and can be bought over-the-counter at natural food stores.

Some women take a few arnica pellets fifteen minutes after birth and continue taking them until they feel its soothing effect. Others carry a topical cream and rub it on the bruised and sore parts of their bodies to lessen the inflammation.

In a situation like Renee and Abigail's, in those vital first moments after delivery, the hospital would bring in all the technology that, frankly, is the reason women have their babies in the hospital. The story is pretty amazing nonetheless if you're talking about that cellular bond between a mom and her baby. All Renee had to do is call to her baby and, after nine months of hearing Mom's voice every day, it was a sound that Abigail sparked to.

In those first moments out of the womb, Abigail, like all babies, was a complicated mix of distinct yet dependent. She needed that cord that connected her to her mother to help her survive until she took her first breath, but once that cord was cut, she was a being of her own. Yet she was so vulnerable. There was no way she could survive without constant care. Fortunately everything she needed to survive she could get from her mom. She needed to stay warm, which she could get by snuggling between her mother's breasts. Abigail also had to be protected from the bacteria of the world she suddenly found herself in. Thankfully she could get that from colostrum, the fluid that preceded her mother's breast milk.

Renee needed Abigail too. Breast-feeding and the skin-to-skin contact between mother and baby produced oxytocin in Renee, which helped her uterus to contract and expel the placenta. This enmeshment puts mom on a high and helps to prevent postpartum depression. Both Renee and Abigail, like all mothers and babies, were extremely sensitive in those precious first moments when Abigail entered the world. By holding on to each other, they bonded. They fulfilled that second requirement the baby has when first emerging from mom; they started to trust each other.

The whole process is so effortless and natural that, left to her own baby intelligence, Abigail probably would have done much of it by herself. In a fascinating study done in Sweden in the early 1990s, moms were asked to lay their newborns on their chests and just wait to see what they did. The researchers filmed the babies, who like all undrugged newborns were alert with eyes wide open, as they oriented themselves to life. They looked around, smacked their lips, and wiggled their way toward their mother's breasts and started to nurse.

Karen Strange has pointed out that far from being unable to see, as doctors thought previously, newborn babies have a vision range of eight to ten inches. Why, that's the perfect distance to look their moms in the eye while they nurse! What a perfect design to keep the mom bonded to her baby so she can feel the glory of this new responsibility and to keep the baby looking at and depending on the best person in the world to make her feel safe and secure.

This scene is a great distance from the way we are trained to think of what happens to babies right after birth, right? Don't they have to be placed on a table away from mom and evaluated to make sure they've got fingers and toes and all parts are in working order?

Well, no, actually they don't.

Pre- and perinatal childbirth educator Karen Strange believes the focus in the labor and delivery room is way out of whack. We're focused mainly on the mom, ignoring the fact that the baby has just completed the journey of his life. That wiggle down the birth canal was tough and took a long time. The poor, defenseless baby gets pulled out into the glaring lights of the delivery room, rubbed with rough towels, jostled onto the table, and generally treated as if he were unable to feel what is being done to him. It's the very definition of a rude awakening. Karen, who is also a midwife and a neonatal resuscitation instructor, sees the way babies are treated as shocking and disturbing.

In maternity wards where the traditional idea of postpartum care prevails, bonding is the second priority. When the baby emerges and starts to take her first breaths, the nurses suction out her mouth and nose to ensure all amniotic fluid is gone. They take her to a warmed examining table where she is evaluated on the Apgar scale. This scale gives her scores for her breathing strength, heart rate, muscle tone, reflexes, and color. This is why you might be alarmed to see the staff holding your baby by the arms and dropping her back on the examining table. That's how they check muscle tone and reflex.

They take this test at one minute of age and at five minutes after birth. The purpose of the score is solely to determine the need for resuscitation in the first minutes of life. This is not the SAT. The test is subjective. One caregiver might rate your baby higher on the ten-point scale than another. Very few babies get a perfect score, so don't stress about how they rank your baby. Unless there is something wrong with her, she'll be doing fine on all these measurements within a few minutes.

Routine Procedures for the Newborn

Procedures vary from institution to institution and in different geographical areas. At birth centers, most procedures are performed on the mother's bed. The following is a rundown of what is typically done to the baby after she is born.

(continued)

Bulb-suctioning. Your baby is typically bulb-suctioned by the doctor at birth and sometimes again by the nurse when she cleans the baby off with a towel. The doctor will use a bulb syringe to remove mucus from your baby's nose and mouth. (The baby is normally not put up on the mother's chest unless delivered by midwives.) Upon your request, some doctors and midwives may be willing to refrain from routinely bulb-suctioning your baby unless absolutely necessary. Aside from being an unpleasant first sensation, excessive bulb-suctioning can interfere with the baby's ability to latch and breast-feed.

The umbilical cord is clamped and cut. You can request that the cord stops pulsating on its own before being clamped and cut. This provides a more gentle transition for the baby to begin breathing on his own, giving his system a final boost of oxygenated blood from the placenta.

The baby is weighed and measured. If this cannot be done in your room, you can request that the nurse wait until after you've had sufficient time to bond with and breast-feed your baby.

The baby is given newborn medications. These almost always consist of a vitamin K injection and erythromycin drops in the eyes. If you don't want your newborn to receive the injection or antibiotics, some institutions will offer a waiver. They can typically be refused if you don't have risk factors and you discuss it with your pediatrician. But in states where these medications are legally mandated, hospitals are generally reticent about offering waivers. If you decide to refuse the vitamin K injection, you can give your baby oral vitamin K drops at home instead. These drops can be ordered online before the birth and will spread out the dosage over a longer period of time. In some places an initial injection of hepatitis B vaccine is also given, so be sure to let the staff know if you'd like to forgo this vaccination at birth. (Hepatitis B is only contracted through contact with blood and bodily fluids, which of course is unlikely for a newborn.)

The baby is bathed. In most settings the parents are given time to bond with the baby after all this is done, and the bath is saved for an hour or more later. However, in some hospitals the baby is taken immediately to the bath. One of the big problems with this practice is that the baby is often cold after being bathed and then has to spend more time separated from the mother, placed under the radiant warmer. Ask if the hospital can wait before bathing your baby so you have time to bond in those first few crucial moments.

Next the baby is injected with vitamin K, which will protect the baby in cases of rare blood disorders. Then they smear her eyes with an antibiotic gel that prevents infection in case you've picked up a nasty case of gonorrhea while you've been pregnant. Insulting, right? About 5 percent of the time women have a case of the clap and don't know about it.

At the same time that your baby is being worked over on the exam table, the nurses may give you a shot of Pitocin that will help the uterus contract sharply to deliver the placenta. Depending on how the birth has gone, you may need some other special care. If you had an episiotomy or a natural vaginal tear, the doctor or midwife will be sewing you up.

As Karen Strange says, why is everyone in such a hurry? Why can't we all just pause for a moment and let the baby adjust to the fact that he's someplace wholly unfamiliar? Left on his own for a moment or two so he can absorb his new world in his own time and integrate what has just happened to him, which is a lot, he will start to wiggle his way up to nurse. Instead, as Abby felt at her C-section, it's like the SWAT team descends. Nils Bergman, the neonatologist who made the film *Kangaroo Mother Care*, says that at birth the brain has two critical sensory needs, smell and touch, and these connect directly to the amygdala. Skin-to-skin contact helps in establishing breast-feeding with newborns.

Even if birth has you overwhelmed and they're sewing you up, you want the baby with you. Ask that they do some of these assessments while the baby is lying on your chest so both of you can get the benefit of the skin-to-skin contact. If you've had a C-section or some other complication in labor, your partner can provide the skin-to-skin contact. It's not quite the same as the baby being on your chest, but it's much better than no contact at all.

The reason it's more important for the baby to be attached to you than to your partner is that during those precious first moments after birth, you are forming a bond that will sustain you during the difficult first months of caring for the baby.

This bond isn't just sentimental; it's a complex hormonal attachment that has a power and rhythm of its own.

The forces that allowed you to birth your baby were stimulated by the oldest and wisest part of your brain, the mammalian part that needs to be shielded from lights and words in order to work its best. To push the baby out of you when you are in this distant, primitive state takes a surge of adrenaline. When that adrenaline is spent, so are you. You're exhausted and the sight and touch of your baby on your chest brings you back.

The baby can sense the location of your nipple, which emits a subtle odor and is a few degrees different in temperature than the rest of your skin. This is why there should be no overpowering scents or chemicals used in the room where you give birth. There are many videos on the Web that show unmedicated newborns who, left to their own instincts in their own time, will gradually make their way to the mother's breast, the left breast in particular.

When your baby attaches to the nipple, his suckling releases a complex rush of hormones that protect you and him, that forge your lifelong bond. Just his first draws on the nipple will help to contract your uterus to inhibit hemorrhaging, as well as stimulate oxytocin, the love hormone, which helps the placenta detach and the uterus to contract. When the hospital staff tries to be helpful in that medical way, they inject you with synthetic oxytocin—in the form of Pitocin—to accomplish the same thing. The synthetic version inhibits the production of the real thing, however, and you might advise the staff you prefer the stuff you make on your own.

In addition to oxytocin, that first attachment at the breast engages the receptors in the breast that signal it to release milk through producing the hormone prolactin. The bond created at that moment has several other layers besides the satisfaction of being able to nourish your child. This simple activity also increases endorphins, what Michel Odent calls the "habit forming hormones," and dopamine, the hormone that helps you cope with pain.

The Postpartum Doula

We're such a culture of individualists that we chide ourselves for not being very robust if something comes along that we can't do on our own. In this category fall women who are convinced they don't need any help when they come home from the hospital with their newborns. In earlier times when you had a baby, members of the village would tend to you for weeks. More recently, many women have their mothers come to stay with them. If you ain't got a village and your mom is otherwise engaged (or you don't want her around), do yourself a huge favor and hire a postpartum doula.

When you get home from the hospital, you'll be exhausted and your adrenaline will still be running very high. You could be happy, elated even. Or you could be sad and overwhelmed. Or all of it in the space of an hour.

"I spend a lot of time talking with a mom about the real truth of motherhood, which is not all pink and gold and Sundays in the park," said Diana Antonelli, a postpartum doula in New York City, describing her initial visit with a postpartum mom. "You're supposed to be so happy. You wanted this for so long and love this baby so much and it's alarming if you are not just over the moon. I tell them it's all part of motherhood and you are going to worry for the rest of your life, so get used to it now."

Besides validating your feelings and helping you trust your instincts, a postpartum doula soothes your physical self. She makes sure you are eating and drinking. She helps with breast-feeding. Diana makes meals for the mom that are rich in vitamins and nutrients like iron to help her repair her body and replenish her for breast-feeding.

Moms who are recovering from C-sections need extra care, Diana said. The combination of labor and surgery and all the drugs makes them especially delicate. "They need to know that it gets better every day. They feel

(continued)

very vulnerable and scared that they can't get up quickly to get to the baby. Physical pain and fear are really difficult when you are a new mom, so the care just steps up a notch or two. Make sure she naps and is eating. Show her the nursing positions that are more comfortable."

Diana gives the C-section moms foot and leg massages to help them work out all the extra fluid from the C-section. "It gets me closer to the new mom and it allows them to let go. It feels good and gets them back into their own body."

What you don't want is for the hospital to take your baby away from you and stick her in with a big bunch of other babies in a nursery. Dr. Marsden Wagner calls placing babies in nurseries "the biggest pediatric mistake in the last hundred years." He's not with his mom, who can keep him warm and make him feel safe, all the while bathing him in protective energy and antibodies.

Makes you wonder who designed this method of caring for a newborn. As Dr. Odent questions, who designed these hospital maternity beds? They are high and thin, discouraging moms from using them to snuggle with their babies. So partially by habit and definitely by design, moms contradict their instinct and hand their babies off to be warehoused, stored in a plastic bin in a big, impersonal room, because the experts say they might do them some harm.

Keeping the baby such a distance away also interferes with the start of breast-feeding, which can be pretty tricky to get started for a first baby. You do not want the nurses feeding your baby with a bottle if you plan to breast-feed. The bottle is a much easier way for the hungry baby to get fed, so she may end up preferring it. If she's not stimulating your breast milk with her demands to be fed, it's going to be harder for you to produce the milk she needs. Ideally, you want to have your baby in a hospital that allows rooming in, meaning that the baby will be with you in a little bed right next to yours and you can reach over and touch her or just look at her anytime you want. Most likely you'll be doing that all the time.

Postpartum Distress Signals

Talk to your medical professional if you experience any of these symptoms:

- You have trouble getting to sleep, and when you do sleep you are awakened by frightening dreams.
- You have trouble completing anything and have become unusually disorganized.
- You are distracted and are having frequent mishaps and accidents.
- You have unusual weight loss or weight gain.
- You are self-medicating with drugs or alcohol.
- You feel hopeless or panicky; you experience extreme mood swings.
- You think of harming yourself or your baby.
- You are withdrawn socially.
- You are crying uncontrollably.
- You're neglecting self-care. You no longer bathe, comb your hair, or brush your teeth.

So let's take this out of the clunky vocabulary of science and back to the intoxicating work of emotion. You are feeding and protecting your baby with that first suckle at the breast, through the warmth of your body, the reassuring gaze into his eyes, and the bath of antibodies and intestinal flora that will prevent the dirty world from messing with his fragile system. He's paying you back by helping you get your body back into prenatal shape by stopping the blood loss and helping the uterus retract and washing away the pain. He's protecting you from getting pregnant again, preventing you from being absorbed in or drained by things that could sap your energy, so that you can protect him. This habit he's helping you form is emotionally and physically satisfying; it drenches you with the feeling of a powerful wordless connection. Together you and your baby have created your own vibrant world of interconnectivity and dependence.

Epilogue

Since releasing our documentary, *The Business of Being Born*, and while writing *Your Best Birth*, we have been flooded with stories of women and men who have "awakened" to the message that something is terribly wrong with the way our culture treats childbirth. The stories that pour into our Web site are alternately heartbreaking and uplifting. They frequently move us to tears. The one recurring story we hear over and over is from the woman who realized *after* her first birth that she needed to be much more informed and proactive for the second one. Many times this second birth is an opportunity for personal growth and often heals the psychological wounds from the first one. But with over one-third of first-time mothers giving birth by C-section, it will soon be more difficult for those mothers to choose another route the next time around.

Women are already driving over state lines and laboring in hospital parking lots in order to have a VBAC. It will only become harder for women to find a provider or a hospital that offers VBAC, and we may see a future where all women are forced into repeat surgeries for subsequent births. Having visited private hospitals in Brazil with C-section rates over 90 percent, we can tell you that this is not science fiction. This could become the norm in the United States as well. Remember, midwives used to be the norm in this country (well, everywhere) and now they are considered alternative. So, it's not inconceivable that a few more policy changes could alter the landscape of birth even more radically.

But as the system keeps pushing women toward more medicalized births, it's inspiring to see a new generation of parents and obstetricians pushing back. Midwives all over the country have reported that demand for their services is growing. Some home birth midwives told us that their clients have doubled since our film was released in 2008. Medical students and nursing students are demanding rotations in midwifery and more training in the physiological process of birth. The system has swung so far out of control that attitudes are shifting back toward respect for the natural process. The same trends are happening with the environment, as "going green" is becoming a part of mainstream culture. So it makes sense that transforming our birth culture should reflect this growing consciousness about the negative effects of technology and industrialization.

Something has got to give, and in our for-profit health care system that means consumers need to speak with their pocketbooks. After reading this book, we hope that you will begin to demand more choices in childbirth in your community. If your health insurance company will not cover midwives or home births, then switch companies and let them know why. If you work for a big corporation, then tell your employer that their plan should cover midwifery and home birth. If you used a fantastic OB-GYN or midwifery practice, tell other women to seek them out. If you had a negative experience, warn others. If your local hospital doesn't have a birth center or offer midwifery services, make a big fuss about it. We need to start lifting the veil on this issue because our failure to normalize birth will impact future generations in ways that we cannot even imagine. One simple action you can take is to participate in the birth survey sponsored by the Coalition for Improving Maternity Services (CIMS) at www.thebirthsurvey.com.

Many parents are starting to understand that the birth of their child is something that can be "taken away" from them. It takes a lot of research and guidance to make sure you are with providers who will respect your family's birth plan. Today, there is a sad disconnect between a "safe" birth and an "empowered" birth, as if you needed to give up one to achieve the other. But we can't just be in the business of delivering "perfect" babies and ignoring the mother's experience. We have to start investing in mothers' journeys as well.

At the end of the day, we feel that the true mark of a "best birth" is when the mother is respected, informed, and treated as a participant in every decision about her pregnancy, labor, and delivery. We have observed that when doctors and midwives treat mothers as active participants in their own childbirths, the mothers always feel empowered, no matter whether their births are natural or surgical. And when women feel safe and empowered around their own births, they are able to bond with their babies and enter motherhood from a place of strength and security. We have a long way to go toward making this a reality for every expectant mother, but through sharing information that will support women through this journey, we are moving closer. Our babies will thank us.

Acknowledgments

As in raising a child, it definitely "took a village" to write this book, and we are so thankful for the many experts and families who shared their wisdom and their birth stories with us. Huge thanks to Andrea Barzvi for getting us pregnant and to Danelle Morton for riding out a short and intense labor. Thanks to our team at Grand Central Publishing and our editor, Natalie Kaire, for expertly guiding us through from conception to delivery. We could not have completed the book without the contributions and professional guidance of Eugene Declercq, PhD; Stuart Fischbein, MD; Carolyn Havens Niemann, CNM; Peggy O'Mara; and Maria Iorillo, CPM. Thanks to Ina May Gaskin for generously sharing her knowledge, to Jacques Moritz, MD, for his ongoing support, and to Ana Paula Markel for being a true birth goddess. Thank you to all the amazing women in this book who trusted us with their personal stories. Thanks to Paulo Netto for our beautiful cover photo and to Wendy Shanker for her comedic enhancements. Most of all, thanks to our beautiful boys, Milo, Owen, and Matteo, for the gift of their births.

Appendix

Making Your Birth Plan

Some people advise that you get your birth plan down to one page of general instructions because if you hand the hospital staff a small binder where everything is detailed down to the type of scented candle you prefer, you've basically lost their support. Sounds good to us, along with the recommendation that you tell them how much you like their hospital and how happy you are to be there and state your intention to be flexible when circumstances change.

That's not the type of birth plan we're working here, however. This is more like a birth inventory that will get you to clarify your thinking about what you want so you can make some fundamental decisions about where you want to give birth and who you want around you.

There are many thought-provoking sample birth plans online. Just Google "birth plan" and you'll find some. Much of what follows was inspired by Victoria Macioce-Stumpf's "Birth Plan Organizer" at www .choicesinchildbirth.com. It is recommended that you make sure your name is at the top of your plan, along with your due date and the name of your doctor and/or midwife and doula, if you are using one. Most also have a space for you to list your fears and concerns. If you work with a doula or midwife, she will probably suggest specific guidelines to you as you create your birth plan. Of course, make sure your birth team understands your birth plan, if your doctor is someone you are just meeting for the first time.

The First Stage of Labor

Environment

Wear your own clothes or a hospital gown?

Dim the lights?

Music or silence?

Is privacy important to you? Do you want the door closed or the curtain drawn at all times?

Support

Do you want your partner to be present during all stages of labor and birth?

Can other family members and friends be present?

Do you want to allow medical students or other trainees in or do you want to limit the number of people permitted in your room?

Are doulas allowed? Are they allowed to remain with you during all stages of labor?

Is this place midwife-friendly?

Mobility

Would you like to be able to move freely during labor?

Would you like to be able to use the bath or the shower?

Are IVs standard? Can you opt for a Hep-Lock instead of a standard IV?

Vaginal Exams

Would you like vaginal exams to be limited?

Would you like them done only by nurses or doctors rather than students or residents?

Food and Fluids

Would you like to be able to eat and drink as much as you desire?

Do you want an IV for hydration or not?

Electronic Fetal Monitoring

Do you want continuous monitoring?

Would you prefer it to be intermittent via external auscultation or with a handheld Doppler?

If you want intermittent monitoring, make sure you've chosen a place that allows it.

Induction

Do you prefer not to be induced?

If you are induced, would you only want natural methods? Find out if the hospital uses Cervidil and Cytotec.

What are your feelings about having the bag of waters broken?

Pain Relief

Would you like to handle pain through natural means such as baths and showers?

Would you like coaching from the staff and your partner and/or doula and midwife that includes guiding you to change positions, using a birth ball, massage, breathing, acupressure, visualization, and alternating heat and cold?

Would you like medications and narcotics not to be offered to you?

Under what conditions would you like an epidural?

The Second Stage of Labor

Positions

Do you want your choice of positions?

Do you want to be able to use the squatting bar?

Do you not want to be on your back?

Do you not want your feet in the stirrups?

Pushing

Do you prefer directed pushing or spontaneous bearing down?

Do you want no time limit on pushing?

Do you want prolonged breath holding with guidance from the nurse or staff?

Perineum

Do you want an episiotomy or would you prefer a natural tear?

Do you want the staff to offer you warm compresses or massages on the perineum?

If you prefer an episiotomy, do you want local anesthetic?

The Third Stage of Labor: After the Baby Is Born

Birth

Do you want your partner to cut the cord, not the doctor or nurse?

Do you want your baby placed on you immediately?

Do you prefer the baby to be cleaned up and checked out, then returned to you?

Do you want to save the cord blood?

Breast-Feeding

As soon as the baby is ready, do you want to try to breast-feed?

If you and your baby are separated, do you not want formula offered?

Do you not want artificial nipples (bottles or pacifiers) to be offered?

Newborn Care

Do you want the baby to stay with you at all times unless there is an emergency?

Do you want to delay weighing, measuring, and ointment in eyes until after your recovery period of at least an hour?

Do you want your baby to room with you?

You will be able to meet this challenge! Keep an image of success in your mind. And, remember, when it comes to any of these things, you can change your mind.

Making Your Wishes Known

Let's say you absolutely intend not to have an epidural, but you're not confident about home birth and don't like the birth center in your area. Also your partner and your mother are convinced that the only safe place is the hospital, which doesn't have midwives. You want to find a doctor and a hospital that will support your idea of the birth. So after working through your birth plan, you set out to find the doctor. When you tell her that you are firm in your desire not to have an epidural, she places a hand lightly on your shoulder and tells you all the moms say that at your stage in pregnancy, but almost all of them end up with epidurals.

That's an interesting moment in your decision making for the birth. Do you think she's right? Do you change your firm position to one that she feels is more realistic, based on her experience? Maybe you then decide you should be more open to that idea. Or do you think she's simply not the doctor you want to have at your birth?

You know that hospital staff can get their backs up about a woman armed with a birth plan (which should be a red flag for you about this hospital anyway), so when you go on your tour of a local hospital, you're not going to go there clutching your plan in your hand. You have the main points of it pretty well fixed in your head because you and your partner (and maybe your doula or midwife) have worked it through carefully. You agree you want to wear your own nightgown, not a hospital gown, and you want your partner to be in the delivery room as well as your doula. You also want to move around when you're in labor to help the baby progress because you are still convinced that you don't want an epidural.

The birth plan is not inflexible, but it is a tool that can clarify what you want and help you find people who will support you and a place where you have a better chance of getting the birth that you feel most satisfied with.

A Simple Birth Plan

Once you've decided on your birth plan, it's easy to reduce what you want to one page. Follow the same heading for the page of this simplified plan, including your name, your partner's name, caregiver, due date, and a brief pleasant introduction. Then you can simply list the things you wish to avoid in this birth. Most hospitals should be familiar enough with birth plans by now to respond to a basic list. It might be as simple as listing:

We wish to avoid:

Medication
Shaving
Enemas
IV unless Hep-Lock is available
Stripping of membranes
Breaking of waters
Pitocin or other labor-induction methods
Lying down for pushing
Episiotomy
Forceps or vacuum extraction
Bottle feeding

We wish to include:

My own nightgown for the birth
Our own music selection
Non-narcotic pain relief
My partner, mom, and doula
Massage
Water birth

Resources for Your Best Birth

Midwives

American College of Nurse-Midwives
  www.acnm.org; www.midwife.org
Better Birth America
  www.betterbirthamerica.com
Birth Partners
  birthpartners.com
Canadian Association of Midwives (CAM)
  canadianmidwives.org
Childbirth and Postpartum Professional
  Association of Canada (CAPPA Canada)
  cappacanada.ca
Citizens for Midwifery
  cfmidwifery.org
Midwifery Today
  www.midwiferytoday.com
Midwives Alliance of North America (MANA)
  mana.org
MyBirthTeam
  www.mybirthteam.com
MyMidwife.org

Doulas

Association of Labor Assistants and Childbirth Educators
(ALACE)
(888) 222-5223
www.alace.org
Childbirth and Postpartum Professional Association
www.cappa.net
Doula Network
www.doulanetwork.com
Doulas of North America
(888) 788-DONA (3662)
www.dona.org

Consumer Advocacy and Birth Resources

American Association of Birth Centers (AABC)
www.birthcenters.org
Better Birth America
www.betterbirthamerica.com
The Big Push for Midwives
www.thebigpushformidwives.org
The Birthing Project
(888) 657-9790
www.birthingprojectusa.com
BirthNetwork National
(888) 452-4784
www.birthnetwork.org
Birth Policy: The Big Push for Midwives
www.birthpolicy.org
Birth Works
(888) TOBIRTH
www.birthworks.org

Childbirth.org
 www.childbirth.org
Childbirth Connection
 (212) 777-5000
 www.childbirthconnection.org
Choices in Childbirth
 (212) 983-4122
 www.choicesinchildbirth.org
Citizens for Midwifery
 (888) CFM-4880
 www.cfmidwifery.org
Coalition for Improving Maternity Services (CIMS)
 (888) 282-CIMS
 www.motherfriendly.org
Giving Birth Naturally
 www.givingbirthnaturally.com
International Center for Traditional Childbearing (ICTC)
 (503) 460-9324
 www.blackmidwives.org
My Birth Team
 www.mybirthteam.com
National Advocates for Pregnant Women
 (212) 255-9252
 www.advocatesforpregnantwomen.org
National Latina Institute for Reproductive Health
 (212) 422-2553
 www.latinainstitute.org
National Women's Health Information Center
 (800) 994-9662; (888) 220-5446 TDD
 (telecommunications device for the deaf)
 www.4Woman.gov
Our Bodies Ourselves
 (617) 245-0200
 www.ourbodiesourselves.org
 www.ourbodiesourblog.org

Perinatal Education Associates
www.birthsource.com
SisterSong: Women of Color Reproductive
Health Collective
(404) 756-2680
www.sistersong.net

Childbirth Education

Birthing from Within
(505) 254-4884; (805) 964-6611
www.birthingfromwithin.com
The Bradley Method
(800) 4ABIRTH
www.bradleybirth.com
Henci Goer
www.hencigoer.com
HypnoBirthing
(603) 798-3286
www.hypnobirthing.com
Lamaze International
(800) 368-4404
www.lamaze.org
Sheila Kitzinger, author and birth expert
www.sheilakitzinger.com

Baby-Friendly Hospitals

BFHI USA (Baby Friendly Hospital Initiative in the U.S.)
www.babyfriendlyusa.org/eng/03.html
Unicef: The Baby-Friendly Hospital Initiative (BFHI)
www.unicef.org/programme/breastfeeding/baby.htm

Cesareans

Childbirth Connection
    (212) 777-5000
    www.childbirthconnection.org
International Cesarean Awareness Network, Inc. (ICAN)
    www.ican-online.org
VBAC.com
    (310) 375-3141
    www.vbac.com

Books

The Big Book of Birth, by Erica Lyon
Birth: The Surprising History of How We Are Born, by Tina
    Cassidy
Birth as an American Rite of Passage, by Robbie Davis Floyd, PhD
Birthing from Within, by Pam England, CNM, and
    Rob Horowitz, PhD
Birth Reborn, by Michel Odent, MD
Born in the USA, by Marsden Wagner, MD, MS
The Cesarean, by Michel Odent, MD
Cesarean Voices, published by ICAN
*Childbirth without Fear: The Principles and Practice of Natural
    Childbirth*, by Grantly Dick-Read and Michel Odent
The Complete Book of Pregnancy and Childbirth, by Sheila
    Kitzinger
Creating Your Birth Plan, by Marsden Wagner, MD, and
    Stephanie Gunning
Fearless Pregnancy, by Victoria Clayton, Stuart Fischbein, MD,
    and Joyce Weckl
Gentle Birth Choices, by Barbara Harper and Suzanne Arms
Gentle Birth, Gentle Mothering, by Sarah J. Buckley, MD

A Guide to Effective Care in Pregnancy and Childbirth, by Murray Enkin, Marc J. N. C. Keirse, James Neilson, Caroline Crowther, Lelia Duley, Ellen Hodnett, and Justus Hofmeyr

The Happiest Baby on the Block, by Harvey Karp, MD

Having a Baby Naturally, by Peggy O'Mara

Immaculate Deception II: Myth, Magic and Birth, by Suzanne Arms

Ina May's Guide to Childbirth, by Ina May Gaskin

Lady's Hands, Lion's Heart: A Midwife's Saga, by Carol Leonard

Lying-In: A History of Childbirth in America, expanded edition, by Richard W. Wertz and Dorothy C. Wertz

Obstetric Myths vs. Research Realities, by Henci Goer

The Official Lamaze Guide: Giving Birth with Confidence, by Judith Lothian and Charlotte De Vries

Our Bodies, Ourselves: Pregnancy and Birth, by the Boston Women's Health Book Collective

Painless Childbirth: An Empowering Journey through Pregnancy and Childbirth, by Giuditta Tornetta

Pushed: The Painful Truth about Childbirth and Modern Maternity Care, by Jennifer Block

Simple Guide to Having a Baby, by Janet Whalley, Penny Simkin, and Ann Keppler

Spiritual Midwifery, by Ina May Gaskin

The Thinking Woman's Guide to a Better Birth, by Henci Goer and Rhonda Wheeler

Your Amazing Newborn, by Marshall Klaus and Phyllis Klaus

Magazines

Brain, Child
    www.brainchildmag.com
Cookie
    www.cookiemag.com
Midwifery Today
    www.midwiferytoday.com/magazine/
Mindful Mama Magazine
    www.mindfulmamamagazine.com/
Mothering magazine
    www.mothering.com

Videos

Birth Day, produced by Georges Vinaver and Naoli Vinaver Lopez.
Birth Into Being: The Russian Waterbirth Experience, produced
    by Barbara Harper.
Born in the U.S.A., produced by Marcia Jarmel and Ken Schneider,
    PatchWorks films.
The Business of Being Born, by executive producer Ricki Lake and
    director Abby Epstein.
Gentle Birth Choices, produced by Barbara Harper.
The Happiest Baby on the Block, starring Harvey Karp, MD,
    directed by Nina Montee
It's My Body, My Baby, My Birth, produced by Maria Iorillo.
Orgasmic Birth, directed by Debra Pascali-Bonaro.

Breast-Feeding

Breastfeeding Café
   (607) 272-5436
   www.breastfeedingcafe.com
Dr. Jack Newman Online Breastfeeding Resource Center
   www.drjacknewman.com
Human Milk Banking Association of North America
   (919) 861-4530
   www.hmbana.org
Kellymom Breastfeeding and Parenting
   (727) 823-1000
   www.kellymom.com
La Leche League
   (800) LALECHE (for a referral to someone for free
   breast-feeding advice)
   www.llli.org; www.lalecheleague.org
   (Web site lists free local meetings and resources.)
National Women's Health Information Center
   (800) 994-9662
   www.4Woman.gov
Promotion of Mother's Milk, Inc.
   www.ProMom.org
World Health Organization (recommendations)
   www.who.int/child-adolescent-health/en/

Low-Income and Teen Parent Resources

National Advocates for Pregnant Women
    (212) 255-9252
    www.advocatesforpregnantwomen.org
Planned Parenthood
    (800) 230-PLAN (7526)
    www.plannedparenthood.org
What to Expect Foundation
    (212) 712-9764
    www.whattoexpect.org
Women, Infants, and Children Program (WIC)
    (800) WICWINS (refers to local agency)
    www.northwic.org

Intimate Partner Violence

Battered Mothers Resource Fund, Inc.
    (866) 592-7870
    www.batteredmothers.org
Crime Victims Hotline
    (866) 689-HELP
Domestic Violence Hotline
    (800) 621-HOPE
LAMBDA-GLBT Community Services
    (206) 600-4297
    www.lambda.org
National Coalition against Domestic Violence
    (800) 799-SAFE
    www.ncadv.org

Rape, Sexual Assault, and Incest Hotline
(212) 227-3000
Safe Horizon (for victims of crime and abuse)
(800) 621-HOPE (4673)
www.safehorizon.org

Lesbian and Gay Parenting

Children of Lesbians and Gays Everywhere (COLAGE)
(415) 861-5437
www.colage.org/
Family Equality Council
(617) 502-8700
www.familyequality.org
Gay Parent Magazine
(718) 380-1780
www.gayparentmag.com
National Center for Lesbian Rights
(415) 392-6257
www.nclrights.org

Research

Alliance for the Improvement of Maternity Services (AIMSUSA)
(212) 759-5510
www.aimsusa.org/howsafe.htm
Association for Improvements in the Maternity Services (AIMS)
www.aims.org.uk
Centers for Disease Control and Prevention (CDC)
(800) CDCINFO (232-4636)
TTY (888) 232-6348
www.cdc.gov

Childbirth Connection
>   (212) 777-5000
>   www.childbirthconnection.org

The Cochrane Collaboration
>   www.cochrane.org

National Library of Medicine's PubMed Database
>   www.ncbi.nlm.nih.gov/entrez?db=pubmed

Waterbirth

Birthworks
>   (888) TOBIRTH
>   www.birthworks.org

Waterbirth International
>   www.waterbirth.org

Alternative Medicine

American Association of Drugless Practitioners
>   (903) 843-6401
>   www.aadp.net

American Association of Naturopathic Physicians
>   (206) 298-0126
>   Referral number: (206) 298-0125
>   www.naturopathic.org

American Herbalists Guild
>   (770) 751-6021
>   www.americanherbalistsguild.com

American Holistic Health Association
>   (714) 779-6152
>   www.ahha.org

American Holistic Medical Association
>   (703) 556-9245
>   www.holisticmedicine.org

American Naturopathic Medical Association
  (702) 897-7053
  www.anma.com
Associated Bodywork and Massage Professionals
  (303) 674-0859
  www.abmp.com
Holistic Pediatric Association
  (707) 237-5312
  www.hpakids.org
International Chiropractic Pediatric Association
  (610) 565-2360
  www.icpa4kids.com
National Acupuncture and Oriental Medicine Alliance
  (253) 851-6896
  www.acuall.org
National Center for Complementary and
  Alternative Medicine (NCCAM)
  (888) 644-6226
  nccam.nih.gov
The National Institute of Ayurvedic Medicine
  (888) 246-NIAM
  www.niam.com
North American Society of Homeopaths (NASH)
  (206) 720-7000
  www.homeopathy.org

Postpartum Depression

Depressionafterdelivery.com
  www.depressionafterdelivery.com
  (800) 944-4773 (information request line)
Postpartum Support International (PSI)
  www.postpartum.net

Index